PHYSICAL FITNESS

The pathway to healthful living

PHYSICAL FITNESS

The pathway to healthful living

ROBERT V. HOCKEY, Ed.D.

Chairman, Department of Health, Physical Education,
and Athletics, Trinity University,
San Antonio, Texas

FOURTH EDITION

with 107 *illustrations*

The C. V. Mosby Company

ST. LOUIS • TORONTO • LONDON   1981

MOSBY

1906 **75** 1981
YEARS

A TRADITION OF PUBLISHING EXCELLENCE

FOURTH EDITION

Copyright © 1981 by The C. V. Mosby Company

Previous editions copyrighted 1973, 1977

Printed in the United States of America

The C. V. Mosby Company
11830 Westline Industrial Drive, St. Louis, Missouri 63141

Library of Congress Cataloging in Publication Data

Hockey, Robert V
  Physical fitness.

  Includes bibliographies and index.
  1. Exercise.   2. Physical fitness.   I. Title.
[DNLM: 1. Exertion.   2. Gymnastics.   3. Hygiene.
4. Physical fitness.   QT 255 H685p]
RA781.H57   1981   613.7   80-28800
ISBN 0-8016-2216-6

AC/VH/VH 9 8 7 6 5 4 3   02/B/240

Foreword

Dr. Hockey has addressed his text to the concept that given an understanding and appreciation of the vital role of exercise, the thinking citizen will subscribe to regular exercise as a part of his daily routine.

The author has focused, very properly, on the efficiency of the cardiovascular system as basic to the attainment and maintenance of optimal physical fitness. A strong heart, resiliency in arteries and veins, and a profusion of capillaries throughout all tissues—these are the physiological attributes that are far more important than the bulging muscles that the average citizen of today needs less and less.

The novel approach employed by the author involved student participation in alternate lecture and laboratory sessions throughout the semester. The why and how are presented in the classroom, followed in the next session by activity in the gymnasium related to the topic covered in the preceding lecture. Televised lectures presented to large classes increase the efficiency of this part of the instructional program. The size of the laboratory sections is reduced in order to provide the intimate experiences conducive to effective learning. The comprehensive and pertinent subject matter thereby presented develops progressively that body of knowledge that provides the academic and scientific basis for participating in regular physical activity. It is designed to encourage each student to subscribe to a judiciously self-prescribed program of exercise throughout his lifetime.

The program has been successfully initiated as evidenced by requests from college students for activity periods designed to provide them the opportunity to work out periodically throughout the week, after they have completed the course.

It may be appropriate to risk conjecture at this point in stating that the physical education programs that have developed this type of educational experience for their students will long survive—whether the physical education courses are required or elective. This type of approach may prove equally as desirable in the secondary and elementary schools.

The author is to be commended for the timely and scholarly contributions he has made to a phase of physical education in which academic support has been greatly needed.

Dr. Rico Zenti

*Retired Chairman, Department of Health,
Physical Education, and Recreation,
Northern Michigan University*

Preface

Physical education programs in the past have had as one of their major objectives the development of skill in one or more sports. Skills have been taught and students have been given an opportunity to participate in these sports during the required physical education classes. It was assumed that participation in these sports would be sufficient to develop and maintain an adequate level of physical fitness. It was also assumed that sports participation would become part of the daily living pattern of a great majority of these students later in life. The validity of both of these assumptions appears to be questionable. Despite the fact that there has been an increase in the amount of leisure time, people do not take the time to engage in a regular activity program. They lack sufficient motivation to make time available for this. This could be because the health benefits that can be derived from regular participation in a well-designed physical fitness program have not been emphasized. If people can clearly see advantages that can be derived from such a program, they are more likely to be motivated to participate on a regular basis.

This material is presented in the hope that all individuals might evaluate their present level of physical fitness, might consider carefully all the information available, and then make a wise decision with regard to the importance of physical activity in their lives. Increased knowledge will not contribute to the development of physical fitness, but once individuals are convinced as to the importance of this, then they may have sufficient motivation and sufficient information as to the procedures that they must follow. By careful evaluation of the material presented, a more systematic and intelligent approach to exercise may be possible.

During the past several years, many universities across the country have emphasized this academic content associated with health and physical education. Classes have been organized so that this information could be presented to the students. These classes have been referred to as "Fundamentals of Physical Education," "Basic Movement," "An Academic Approach to Physical Education," and "Foundations of Physical Education." Many of these classes have been organized so that the lecture material is presented one day and an additional one or two days are spent each week in the gymnasium. The material in this book is designed for use in such a class as this.

I am indebted to many people for assistance in the production of this book. I would like to thank Dennis Hickey, Jerry Morrow, Betsy Gross, and Marilyn Peterson for their valuable assistance in the preparation of the manuscript and Dr. Rico Zenti for writing the Foreword. The photographs were taken by Don Pavloski, and the persons used in these photographs were Shelly Sherman, Debbie Anderson, Tim Furno, Roger Harriman, Darcy Hazel, John Shrolec, and Joyce Barnaby.

The drawings were prepared by Eugene Sinervo. I am also indebted to Betty Pangrazzi, Georgia Horton, Shirley Ruecker, Carol Laituri, Martha Shine, and my wife, Judy, for their efforts in preparing parts of this manuscript.

Robert V. Hockey

Contents

ATTITUDE QUESTIONNAIRE*

Initially, it is important to find out how you feel toward exercise and physical education. Each question should be answered by placing an X in the appropriate column. Be *honest* in your answers, but at the same time try to be objective. This is an anonymous questionnaire, and the results will not in any way influence your final grade for this course.

Age _____ **Sex** _____

Laboratory instructor _____

	Strongly agree	Agree	Undecided	Disagree	Strongly disagree
1. Little learning takes place in physical education.	☐	☐	☐	☐	☐
2. At the college level, physical education classes contribute little and do not justify the time and money spent on them.	☐	☐	☐	☐	☐
3. Physical education classes should be offered at the college level, but it should be the student's decision as to whether he takes them or not	☐	☐	☐	☐	☐
4. Most information relative to exercise and physical fitness is common knowledge.	☐	☐	☐	☐	☐
5. Physical education should consist of only those activities that are fun to participate in.	☐	☐	☐	☐	☐
6. I would take physical education classes only if they were a university requirement.	☐	☐	☐	☐	☐
7. Physical education should develop in a student an understanding of the importance of exercise to health and fitness.	☐	☐	☐	☐	☐
8. All required subjects at the college level in all areas except for the area that the student is majoring in should be offered only as electives.	☐	☐	☐	☐	☐
9. Most adults get all the exercise they need by performing their daily tasks.	☐	☐	☐	☐	☐
10. The development of an adequate level of phyical fitness should be a worthwhile objective for all college students.	☐	☐	☐	☐	☐

*Adapted from Corbin, C. B., Dowell, L. J., Lindsey, R., and Talson, M.: Concepts in physical education, Dubuque, Iowa, 1970, Wm. C. Brown Company, Publishers, p. 146.

ACTIVITY INVENTORY*

At the start of the semester it is also important to determine in which activities you participate regularly and in which activities you would like to improve your skill level.

Place a check mark in column 1 next to each activity that you have participated in regularly for at least 8 weeks any time during the past 12 months.

Place a check mark in column 2 next to each activity that you would like to learn more about and in which you would like to increase your skill level.

Numbers are included next to each activity so that computer cards may be used for tabulating results where desired. Students will use the number corresponding to each activity and make their responses next to that number on the IBM card.

Individual and dual sports

	Col. 1	Col. 2
1. Archery	☐	☐
2. Badminton	☐	☐
3. Bowling	☐	☐
4. Calisthenics	☐	☐
5. Fencing	☐	☐
6. Fly casting	☐	☐
7. Golf	☐	☐
8. Gymnastics	☐	☐
9. Handball	☐	☐
10. Hiking	☐	☐
11. Jogging	☐	☐
12. Judo	☐	☐
13. Paddle ball	☐	☐
14. Skating	☐	☐
15. Skiing	☐	☐
16. Tennis	☐	☐
17. Track and field	☐	☐
18. Weight lifting	☐	☐
19. Wrestling	☐	☐

Dance

	Col. 1	Col. 2
20. Ballet	☐	☐
21. Ballroom	☐	☐
22. Creative	☐	☐
23. Folk	☐	☐
24. Square	☐	☐

Team sports

	Col. 1	Col. 2
25. Baseball	☐	☐
26. Basketball	☐	☐
27. Field hockey	☐	☐
28. Ice hockey	☐	☐
29. Soccer	☐	☐
30. Softball	☐	☐
31. Touch football	☐	☐
32. Volleyball	☐	☐

Aquatics

	Col. 1	Col. 2
33. Canoeing	☐	☐
34. Diving	☐	☐
35. Lifesaving	☐	☐
36. Sailing	☐	☐
37. Swimming	☐	☐
38. Water safety instruction (WSI)	☐	☐

Others (list)

	Col. 1	Col. 2
_____	☐	☐
_____	☐	☐
_____	☐	☐
_____	☐	☐

*Adapted from Humphrey, J. H., and Ingram, A. G.: Introduction to physical education for college students, Boston, 1969, Holbrook Press, p. 37.

CHAPTER 1

A new approach to physical education

What do you know about physical education?

T F

☐ ☐ **1.** Physical education activity classes are required in only a small number of universities and colleges.

☐ ☐ **2.** A physically educated person could be defined as one who is physically fit.

☐ ☐ **3.** Most college students have the necessary motivation to participate regularly in some form of physical activity.

☐ ☐ **4.** The main reason many people are not more active is that they do not have sufficient time to exercise.

☐ ☐ **5.** Keeping students occupied and letting them have fun and play games are probably the most important objectives of a good physical education program.

☐ ☐ **6.** More people now appear to be concerned about exercise and fitness than previously were in this country.

☐ ☐ **7.** Gaining knowledge about physical fitness will definitely contribute to an improvement in the level of physical fitness.

☐ ☐ **8.** The human body has experienced little or no difficulty in adapting to increased mechanization in today's society.

Physical education may be defined simply as that integral part of total education that contributes to the development of the individual through some form of physical activity. It must involve a carefully planned sequence of learning experiences designed to fulfill the growth, development, and behavior needs of each student.

PHYSICAL EDUCATION—A REQUIREMENT OR AN ELECTIVE?

Each day thousands of young men and women take part in some organized physical education program—a requirement at many colleges and universities. A survey conducted in 1977 involving 632 four-year universities indicated that 53% of these institutions had a physical education requirement for all students and an additional 13% required it in some departments or colleges. This represented a 17% decrease over the previous 4 years. However, it is interesting to note that 81% of the universities not requiring physical education did not require students to take *any* specific courses. This same survey showed that more than 94% of all institutions provide the opportunity for the general college student to take a variety of physical education classes. This emphasizes the importance placed on physical education at the university level.[8]

Fraleigh and Gustafson[3] indicate that for something to be required, exposure to it is essential to the well-being of those for whom it is required. Many college students lack an understanding of the potential values of participation in physical education activities and believe that physical education is a waste of time and has little to contribute to their total education. The fact that such a large number of universities and colleges require physical education indicates that there is nearly unanimous agreement that physical education does play an important part in the total education of college students.

As freshmen and sophomores, most students find that there are a large number of subjects that must be taken. Many students resent having to take these courses because most of them appear to have little to do with their major areas of specialization. However, these courses are required in an attempt to expose students to the "general" education considered desirable for American youth. For many of them it is probably difficult to understand why so many universities require physical education. This may be an indication that most high school students in the United States have not been exposed to good physical education programs. Certainly this is a generalization; however, if high schools were doing an adequate job training youth in proper physical education skills and knowledge, students would not be asking why they have to take physical education. Also, people would be free of a tremendous number of physical and mental disabilities.[9]

Sanborn and Hartman present some interesting information in support of required physical education. Their results are summarized as follows:

1. Studies among students indicate that they prefer physical education to be required.
2. A large majority of colleges require physical education.
3. Regular physical activity is absolutely necessary as one contributing factor to the health and physical fitness necessary for the pursuit of exacting studies.
4. If it is placed on an elective basis, those who need physical education will *not* elect it.
5. Very few college freshmen can be considered to be physically educated.[10]

IMPORTANCE OF THE ACADEMIC APPROACH TO PHYSICAL EDUCATION

The report of the President's Commission on Higher Education states that "college programs of physical education should provide an opportunity for the student to put into practice his theoretical knowledge of healthful habits."[5] This statement implies that there is a theoretical body of knowledge associated with physical education. Unfortunately, students graduating from high school in most cases have not been exposed to this knowledge. Many high school programs are directed entirely toward the development of sports skills or physical fitness, or both. These are important but should not constitute the entire high school program.

Oseness and Joyce[7] interviewed physical educators, coaches, administrators, and health educators in the state of Kansas with regard to the possible adoption of a new curriculum for high school physical education. The curriculum that was proposed included information relating to the value of physical activity to the human body. It also utilized lecture and laboratory sessions aimed at assisting the student in understanding himself and the benefits that could be derived from physical activity. The results of this study indicate that there is a definite need for such a curriculum change and that the quantity of academic content included in high school physical education programs should be increased. Other positive indications from this study were as follows:

1. It was generally believed that the public would accept such a program.
2. The proposed program had more carry-over potential than the existing program.
3. Only 8% of the 80 high school personnel interviewed indicated that they would *not* be willing to try such a program as this.

Such a change is difficult to initiate and involves much time. During the past 12 years very few high schools have implemented such a program; however, this is not true at the college level. The majority of universities across the country now offer a program designed to acquaint students with knowledge concerning exercise and fitness. This approach has been referred to as an academic approach to physical education.

The fact that such an effort has been made during the past 12 years may explain the added participation and interest in physical fitness during recent years in the United States.

The following objectives are presented in an attempt to identify the information associated with physical education that appears to be important. Each student should (1) acquire knowledge of the structure and functioning of the human body; (2) understand fully the role of exercise in improving one's level of physical fitness so that each can decide how much is necessary and what kind of activity is best; (3) develop an understanding of the physiological benefits that can be derived from regular exercise; (4) understand the principles involved in conducting a good exercise or training program and be able to develop an acceptable program; (5) attain knowledge of the fundamental relationship between exercise, diet, and weight control.

CRITERIA FOR A GOOD PHYSICAL EDUCATION PROGRAM

The American public has been misinformed concerning what constitutes a good physical education program and what values can be attained through regular participation in such a program. Many people still confuse athletics with physical education.

A person who has been exposed to a good physical education program should be able to respond positively to the following questions:

YES NO

☐ ☐ 1. Do you understand how your body functions and the changes that take place as a result of regular exercise?

☐ ☐ 2. Do you understand the effects of various types and intensities of activities on your body?

☐ ☐ 3. Can you design an activity program to meet your present and future needs?

☐ ☐ 4. Do you know how to evaluate your present level of physical fitness? Can you?

☐ ☐ 5. Do you have adequate knowledge and skill in a sufficient number of activities so that you can enjoy participation in these activities throughout all seasons of the year regardless of geographic location or the facilities available?

☐ ☐ 6. Do you understand the values of regular physical activity and particularly its role in maintaining a healthy, more efficient body?

YES NO

☐ ☐ 7. Do you participate regularly in an exercise program designed to develop and maintain an adequate level of physical fitness?

☐ ☐ 8. Do you maintain an adequate level of physical fitness by having a body capable of meeting the daily demands made on it without experiencing undue fatigue?

☐ ☐ 9. Do you demonstrate adequate social adjustment by reacting favorably to such things as winning, losing, adversity, team play, and competition?

☐ ☐ 10. Do you demonstrate a feeling of self-confidence by being aware of your strengths and weaknesses, your abilities and limitations, and by being concerned about your appearance?

The preceding examples give some idea of the philosophies behind certain types of programs that are being developed at the college level and the academic content within these programs. It is apparent that being physically educated is indeed an important part of total education. These programs seek to answer some of the typical questions that frequently are presented at the college level: What is the unique purpose of physical education in the college? What does the program have to offer students that is considered important enough to permit it to continue to assume its present status? Should academic credit be given for physical education at the college level? How these questions are answered will depend on how physical education is perceived. Unfortunately, many persons have an entirely false concept of physical education. As Blackenbury indicates, "The day may be gone when the gym teacher unlocks the door, throws out the ball, and turns his attention to such weightier matters as plotting defensive strategy for the football team."[1] This situation, however, still exists in many of our schools. To a large percentage of adults in this country, physical education means nothing more than "fun and games" for the students. Some physical educators believe that keeping the students

"occupied" is all that is necessary as far as physical education is concerned. A reeducation of many adults, teachers, and students is necessary.

IMPORTANCE OF EXERCISE AND PHYSICAL FITNESS

A recent nation-wide survey indicates that good health is the most important concern of more than 70% of the entire population in the United States.[4] This same report shows that it is the firmly established belief of almost all Americans that if they changed their life-styles, ate more nutritious food, reduced smoking, and exercised regularly, their health would improve tremendously.

The American population has good reason to be concerned about exercise, fitness, and health. The seriousness of this problem can be ascertained after consideration of the following facts:

1. The United States has the highest incidence of cardiovascular disease in the world, with many of these deaths directly associated with obesity and inactivity.

2. More than 60% of the adult population can be considered overweight or obese.

3. The American population spends more than $35 million each year on worthless methods aimed at improving physical fitness or losing weight the easy, "no work" way.[12]

4. Approximately 65% recognize they would be healthier if they changed their eating habits.

5. Less than 40% of the American adult population exercise regularly.

6. Approximately 35% of the population 17 years of age or older smoke regularly.

7. The incidence of low back pain in the U.S. continues to increase. More than 80% of the low back pain problems are caused by improper muscular development.

It is apparent, however, that today more people in the United States are interested in exercise, fitness, and health. This is evidenced by the following information:

1. More people than ever before are exercising regularly.
2. More than 30 million people have stopped smoking.
3. Nutritional habits have changed as the population has become more aware of the nutritional content of foods and the effects of different ingredients.
4. The incidence of heart disease and other cardiovascular disorders has decreased.

It is obvious that it is possible to change attitudes and behavior. The question is how best to influence each specific habit and how to do this most effectively.

Three main reasons for physical inactivity, given by those who recognize that they do not get enough exercise, are insufficient time, lack of self-discipline, and lack of interest. Despite the fact that lack of sufficient time is by far the most frequent answer, these same people usually find time to watch their favorite basketball team, football team, or television program or to engage in some form of "passive" relaxation. It has been estimated that the average American family watches television 5 hours daily. It is no wonder that the American population has been referred to as a "nation of spectators."

Time, obviously, is not the explanation.

People can usually find time to do what they want to do. In recent years there has been a tremendous increase in the amount of leisure time available to each individual. This has come about mainly because of decreased time spent at work. This relationship, showing the trend over the last 50 years, is presented in Fig. 1-1. Whether this increased amount of leisure time is good or not depends on its use. If used as many Americans use it today, in aimless play and in various forms of passive amusement, then it is obviously not good for them or for society. One of the major aims of physical education classes should be to reverse the trend toward physical inactivity and thus to lessen the amount of physical degeneration in our society.

The President's Council suggests several ways of persuading people to exercise regularly: (1) show them how to fit exercise into their busy schedules; (2) convince older people that age is no barrier to exercise; (3) appeal to their concern for health and an attractive appearance; (4) convince them that exercise can be enjoyable; and (5) present more information to them on the types of exercise that are best and the amount of exercise necessary to develop and maintain adequate fitness.[6]

The President's Council on Physical Fitness further suggests the following:

No longer can we afford to consider anyone fully educated until he knows how—and is thoroughly

Fig. 1-1. Decrease in work time and increase in leisure—1920 to 1970. (Adapted from Van Huss, Niemeyer, Olson, and Friedrick.[11])

motivated—to keep himself in the best possible physical condition at all times. Achieving this end for all students should be one of the primary goals of every college.[2]

The existing situation implies that each member of society must choose how this increased leisure time is to be spent. If the stated objectives of physical education are achieved, it is anticipated that more students will be motivated to participate regularly in physical activity. The student who has been exposed to the academic body of knowledge relating to physical education will be in a position to make a much wiser decision when he has a full understanding of the facts.

It also seems to be important in physical education to teach those activities and to encourage students to take those activities that have some carry-over value—the ones that adults can participate in later in life. Blackenbury states:

Man always finds time to do what he wants to do and people tend to enjoy doing the things they do well. If students learn the basic skills essential to good performance, and if they learn them in an atmosphere they find pleasant, it is likely their learning will become the basis for many hours of enjoyment as adults.[1]

Knowledge is very important in changing habits and behavior, yet knowledge alone is not enough. For example, 70% of those who smoke know that regular smoking increases their chances of cancer, yet they still smoke. Two out of every three adults believe that they ought to exercise more than they do. Knowledge, however, is the first step and is certainly an essential component of change.[4]

SUMMARY

Motivation is the key to getting a person to exercise. Simply increasing an individual's knowledge of exercise and physical fitness is not enough; he must change his attitude toward regular exercise. If he believes strongly enough

in physical activity and exercise, he will want to do something about it. For many persons an understanding of the benefits that can be derived from exercise is sufficient motivation for them to engage in some form of regular physical activity. One would hope that as a result of material contained in this book many students will be motivated to devise their own exercise program and make exercise a part of their daily living habits.

REFERENCES

1. Blackenbury, R. L.: Physical education: an intellectual emphasis? Quest, Dec., 1963, p. 3.
2. Fitness and leadership: suggestions for colleges and universities, President's Council on Physical Fitness, Washington, D.C., 1964, U.S. Government Printing Office.
3. Fraleigh, W. P., and Gustafson, W. F.: Can we defend required programs? Journal of Health, Physical Education, and Recreation **35:**32, Feb., 1964.
4. Health maintenance, Newport Beach, Calif., Nov., 1978, Pacific Mutual Life Insurance Co., p. VI.
5. Higher education for American democracy: establishing the goals, President's Commission on Higher Education, New York, 1948, Harper & Brothers, p. 54.
6. Newsletter, President's Council on Physical Fitness and Sports, April, 1976, p. 16.
7. Oseness, W. H., and Joyce, P. J.: An analysis of attitudes toward certain recommended changes in the physical education curriculum. Paper presented at 1969 American Association for Health, Physical Education, and Recreation, Central District Convention, St. Paul, Minn.
8. Oxendine, J. B.: The general instruction program in physical education at four-year colleges and universities: 1977, Journal of Health, Physical Education, and Recreation, **49:**21, Jan., 1978.
9. Penman, K. A.: Physical education for college students, ed. 2, St. Louis, 1968, The C. V. Mosby Co., p. 6.
10. Sanborn, M. A., and Hartman, B.: Issues in physical education, Philadelphia, 1964, Lea & Febiger.
11. Van Huss, W., Niemeyer, R., Olson, H., and Frederick, J.: Physical activity in modern living, ed. 2, Englewood Cliffs, N.J., 1969, Prentice-Hall, Inc., p. 3.
12. Wyden, P., and Wyden, B.: Why diet and exercise fads don't turn your fatness into fitness. In The healthy life, New York, 1966, Time, Inc.

CHAPTER 2

The cardiovascular system and cardiovascular disease

What do you know about the cardiovascular system and cardiovascular disease?

T   F

☐ ☐ **1.** The function of the left side of the heart is to circulate purified blood to all parts of the body.

☐ ☐ **2.** Veins always carry used blood back to the heart.

☐ ☐ **3.** The size of the heart cannot increase with exercise.

☐ ☐ **4.** The purpose of the valves in the circulatory system is to regulate the flow of blood by allowing it to flow in only one direction.

☐ ☐ **5.** People who have desk jobs are more likely to have varicose veins than those who are more active.

☐ ☐ **6.** The force of the heart is largely responsible for the return of blood through veins to the heart.

☐ ☐ **7.** A low resting heart rate is a good indication the heart is not functioning efficiently.

☐ ☐ **8.** A person who has smoked for 5 years cannot reduce his chances of a heart attack by discontinuing this habit.

☐ ☐ **9.** Cholesterol is not essential to the normal functioning of the body.

☐ ☐ **10.** Vigorous exercise is not recommended by physicians for prevention of heart disease.

☐ ☐ **11.** High blood pressure and obesity are positively related.

☐ ☐ **12.** The incidence of heart disease in the United States is greater per 100,000 of population than in any other industrialized country.

Information relating to the construction and function of the heart and circulatory system is presented so that some of the problems associated with heart disease may be better understood.

THE HEART AS A MUSCULAR PUMP

The heart is simply a muscular pump that provides the force necessary to keep the blood circulating throughout the network of arteries. This hollow, muscular organ is located between the lungs and the diaphragm in what is known as the medial sternal space. It is mostly to the left of the midline of the body with its apex pointing down.

It can actually be considered to consist of two pumps. A thick muscular wall known as the *septum* divides the heart cavity down the middle into what is known as a *right heart* and a *left heart*.

On each side is an upper chamber known as the atrium and a lower chamber called the ventricle. Each atrium is separated from the ventricle below by a valve, which regulates the flow of blood.[34] These are referred to as atrioventricular valves.

The *right heart* receives blood that has completed its cycle through the body. This blood collects in the right atrium of the heart. Actually this used blood from the body reaches the heart by two large veins—the superior and inferior venae cavae. The superior vena cava returns blood from the head and the arms while the inferior vena cava drains the blood from the trunk and the legs. A third opening into the right atrium is the coronary sinus. This returns blood that is used by the heart muscle itself. From the right atrium the blood enters the right ventricle through the tricuspid valve. The blood is pumped from the right ventricle through the pulmonary arteries to the lungs, where it picks up fresh oxygen and gives up carbon dioxide. The function of the right heart, then, is to pump blood to the lungs, where oxygen is picked up and carbon dioxide is eliminated. The blood flow associated with the right heart is illustrated in Fig. 2-1, *A*.

The *left heart* receives the reoxygenated

Fig. 2-1. A, Blood flow associated with right heart. Note that major purpose of right heart is to pump blood to lungs, where oxygen is picked up and carbon dioxide eliminated. **B,** Blood flow associated with left heart. Note that left heart is responsible for pumping blood out of left ventricle via the aorta to all parts of body. (Drawings by Eugene Sinervo.)

blood, which is returned through the pulmonary veins.[34] This blood collects in the left atrium and passes from this upper chamber to the lower, through the mitral, or bicuspid, valve. It is this left ventricle that pumps the blood out of the heart. The blood passes through the aorta—the largest artery in the body—to all parts of the body. Fig. 2-1, *B*, illustrates the blood flow associated with the left heart.

VALVES OF THE HEART

The valves play an important role in regulating the flow of blood. Besides the two atrioventricular valves that have been explained previously, two other valves are located where the pulmonary artery and aorta join the ventricles. These valves as well as the two atrioventricular valves are unidirectional and allow blood to flow in only one direction. These prevent the backward flow of blood during diastole, when the heart is relaxed. The heart sounds that may be heard with a stethoscope are caused by the closing of the valves of the heart. The sound that is heard is lubb-dupp. The first of these sounds is caused by the atrioventricular valves as they close when the contraction of the ventricles takes place. At this time the other two valves, the aortic and pulmonary valves, are open as blood is being ejected from the heart. The dupp sound is made by the closing of the valves in the aorta and pulmonary arteries as the heart again is filling with blood.

BLOOD VESSELS

A clear distinction is necessary between arteries and veins. Any vessel taking blood away from the heart is an artery, whereas any vessel returning blood to the heart is a vein. A knowledge of the structure of the artery is most important in understanding heart disease. The cross sections of an artery and vein are compared in Fig. 2-2.[6] Notice that both arteries and veins have three layers: (1) intima, or innermost layer, (2) media, or middle layer, and (3) adventitia, or outer layer. However, the muscular wall of the normal artery is much thicker than

that of the vein. This allows the arteries to be elastic so that when blood is ejected from the heart they can expand to receive the blood. During the relaxation phase of the cardiac cycle, the muscular walls of the arteries then contract to keep the blood moving through the arterial system.

The arterial branches eventually become smaller and smaller. The smallest branches are known as *capillaries*. It is here that the oxygen and nutrients leave the blood and enter the body cells and that carbon dioxide and metabolic wastes leave the cells and are picked up by the bloodstream.

As fatty deposits accumulate on the inner arterial walls, they tend to lose their elasticity and become smaller in size. This decreases the ability of the circulatory system to function efficiently and increases the possibility of cardiovascular problems.

Blood is returned to the heart through the network of veins. As indicated, these veins do not have the thick, muscular walls that most arteries have. For this reason there is less pressure in the veins. This does not create a problem for blood returning from the upper parts of the body, since gravity will assist in the return of this blood to the heart.[32] However, blood in the arms and legs must rely on the squeezing action

Fig. 2-2. Comparison between cross section of an artery and a vein. Note that muscular wall (media) of artery is much thicker than that of vein. (Drawing by Eugene Sinervo.)

of the muscles in order to be returned to the heart. There is a system of valves in the veins that allows the blood to flow only toward the heart. These veins are located between the skeletal muscles, and when the muscles contract, these veins are "squeezed" and the blood flows toward the heart. If too much time is spent standing at attention, it is not uncommon for a person to experience fatigue and to pass out. Blood is not returned from the lower parts of the body to the heart, and it "pools" in these lower areas. Varicose veins result from the failure of used blood to be returned to the heart at a "fast enough" rate. The accumulated blood causes the veins to swell. Varicose veins occur frequently in individuals whose jobs require that they stand for a number of hours each day or who remain seated for extended periods of time.

BASIC TERMS ASSOCIATED WITH THE CARDIOVASCULAR SYSTEM

Certain basic terms associated with the cardiovascular system need to be explained to understand the material that is presented later. These basic terms include (1) heart rate, (2) stroke volume, (3) cardiac output, and (4) blood pressure.

Heart rate

For an average untrained person in a resting position, the heart beats approximately 72 times per minute. This is known as the heart rate, or pulse. It is caused by the impact of the blood on the arteries as the heart contracts. It can be detected easily by placing a finger on the radial artery located on the lateral side of the wrist or at one of the carotid arteries that pass anteriorly in the neck. In children this rate is much faster, whereas in the highly trained individual the heart becomes more efficient, and the resting heart rate is often much lower.*

Stroke volume

Each time the heart contracts, a certain amount of blood is ejected. This is known as the stroke volume, which is defined as the amount of blood ejected with each beat of the heart. In the resting condition for an untrained person the stroke volume is approximately 70 ml.

Cardiac output

The cardiac output is defined as the amount of blood that the heart is able to circulate each minute. It is dependent on the stroke volume and the heart rate.

Cardiac output = Heart rate × Stroke volume

Using the average figures presented previously, the average cardiac output is calculated as follows:

$$\begin{aligned} \text{Cardiac output} &= \text{Heart rate} \times \text{Stroke volume} \\ &= 72 \times 70 \\ &= 5{,}040 \text{ ml/min} \\ &= 5.04 \text{ l./min} \end{aligned}$$

This means that for a person in the resting condition approximately 5 liters of blood are circulated by the heart each minute.*

Blood pressure

Blood pressure is the amount of force that the blood exerts against the artery walls. It is usually expressed in millimeters of mercury and is the force that keeps the blood flowing through the arteries. It is generated by the heart as it contracts and is maintained by the elasticity of the artery walls. Everyone has blood pressure, for without it the blood would not circulate.[21]

Each time the heart contracts, the blood pressure goes up. The contraction phase of the cardiac cycle is defined as systole; thus this upper blood pressure is referred to as the systolic blood pressure. Each time the heart relaxes, the blood pressure decreases. The relaxation phase

---

*These training effects are discussed in detail in Chapter 9.

*A liter (l.) is approximately equivalent to a quart.

Fig. 2-3. Measurement of blood pressure with sphygmomanometer.

Table 2-1. Normal blood pressure for college-age men and women*

Sex	Blood pressure	Mean	Standard deviation
Male	Systolic	123	13.7
Male	Diastolic	76	9.9
Female	Systolic	116	11.8
Female	Diastolic	72	9.7

*From Lasser, R. P., and Master, A. M.: Mean resting blood pressure in apparently healthy persons 20 to 106 years of age, Geriatrics **14:**345, 1959.

off the flow of blood to the forearm, and no heart sound can be heard when a stethoscope is placed on the compressed artery just below the cuff. As the air pressure in the cuff is released, the mercury level drops. Eventually a point will be reached at which the blood pressure in the artery is just greater than the air pressure in the cuff. Blood will now begin to flow through the artery, and the heart sound may be heard by using the stethoscope. This is the systolic or upper pressure—it is the maximum pressure that can be produced by the heart.

As the physician continues to let air out of the cuff, the sounds heard through the stethoscope will become louder as more blood passes through the artery. Finally, a point will be reached at which the distinct heart sounds disappear as the blood is flowing steadily through the artery. At this point the height of the mercury shows the diastolic or lower pressure representing the least amount of pressure in the artery.[21] The average, or normal, blood pressure figures for college-age men and women are presented in Table 2-1.

CARDIOVASCULAR DISEASE

The word *cardiovascular* refers to the heart and blood vessels that make up the lifestream of the human body. Diseases affecting this system may be inherited, can result from various living

of the cardiac cycle is referred to as diastole, and hence the lower blood pressure is known as diastolic blood pressure. Blood pressure is written as systolic/diastolic. For example, 120/80 indicates that the systolic blood pressure is 120 mm of mercury while the diastolic blood pressure is 80 mm.

In measuring blood pressure, the physician uses a sphygmomanometer (Fig. 2-3). An airtight cuff is wrapped around the arm just above the elbow. The cuff is connected to a glass tube filled with mercury. Air is pumped into the cuff by squeezing a bulb. As the cuff becomes tighter, it compresses a large artery in the arm—the brachial artery. This temporarily cuts habits, or can be caused by infection or injury.

The major cause of cardiovascular disease is the buildup of fatty substances along the inside walls of blood vessels. These blood vessels then narrow to create a condition known as atherosclerosis. The result is that blood may not be supplied in sufficient quantity to various parts of the body, and these areas are thus deprived of a sufficient supply of oxygen.

The heart, which is comprised of muscular tissue, also requires its own continuous blood supply. This supply is delivered through a special set of arteries known as the coronary arteries.

Damage may occur to the heart itself, in the coronary arteries, or in the other blood vessels throughout the body. Cardiovascular disease is thus not a single disease but includes a number of specific diseases.

Each year more than 40 million Americans are afflicted with some form of cardiovascular disease. The estimated prevalence of the major cardiovascular diseases is presented in Fig. 2-4.

The leading causes of death in the United States in 1977 are summarized in Fig. 2-5. These data clearly show that cardiovascular dis-

eases claim more lives than all other causes of death combined, accounting for more than 52% of all deaths.

The breakdown of deaths by the major types of cardiovascular disorders is presented in Fig. 2-6. Heart attacks account for approximately 65% of all cardiovascular diseases, while the percentage attributable to strokes is slightly less than 19%.[19]

The cost attributed to heart and blood vessel diseases in this country has been estimated at more than $40 billion, in addition to lost income, and an estimated loss of 50 million mandays of production for the year 1980.

Probably the most alarming factor, however, is that the incidence of death from cardiovascular disease in the United States is higher than in any other country in the world. The annual mortality rates for deaths from atherosclerotic heart disease for certain selected countries are presented in Fig. 2-7. These figures are based on the annual mortality rate per 100,000 of the total population, both male and female.

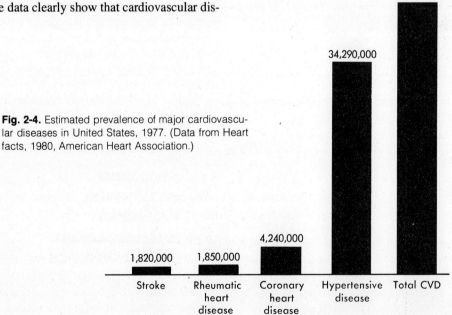

Fig. 2-4. Estimated prevalence of major cardiovascular diseases in United States, 1977. (Data from Heart facts, 1980, American Heart Association.)

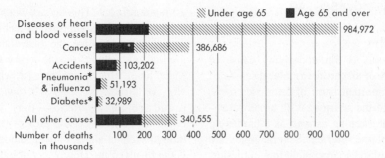

Fig. 2-5. Leading causes of death in United States, 1977. (Data from Heart facts, 1980, American Heart Association.)

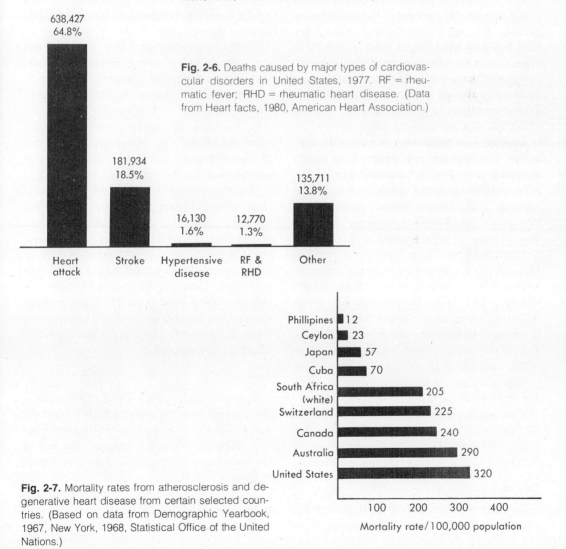

Fig. 2-6. Deaths caused by major types of cardiovascular disorders in United States, 1977. RF = rheumatic fever; RHD = rheumatic heart disease. (Data from Heart facts, 1980, American Heart Association.)

Fig. 2-7. Mortality rates from atherosclerosis and degenerative heart disease from certain selected countries. (Based on data from Demographic Yearbook, 1967, New York, 1968, Statistical Office of the United Nations.)

COMMON CARDIOVASCULAR DISEASES

Atherosclerosis

Atherosclerosis is the underlying cause of more than 95% of all cardiovascular diseases. It is the more important form of arteriosclerosis, or hardening of the arteries. With atherosclerosis there is a thickening as well as a hardening of the walls of the arteries. Several lipids are present in the bloodstream, including cholesterol, triglyceride, phospholipids, and fatty acids. It is believed that atherosclerosis usually begins with a deposit of some form of fatty material on the inner layer of the arterial wall. Such a deposit is known as a plaque. After a time these deposits may become embedded within the inner layer of the artery—the intima. The lumen, or opening, through which the blood must pass gradually narrows with each deposit, and the blood flow may be seriously impaired.[9]

Atherosclerosis may begin at an early age, and yet the symptoms may not appear until middle age or later. Sanders[28] indicates that "a fact often overlooked by the public is that almost everyone in the United States over the age of twelve has atherosclerosis to some degree." This appears to be supported in a study by Enos, Holmes, and Beyer,[9] who examined 300 United States soldiers killed in action during the Korean War. The average age of these soldiers was only 22.1 years. Despite this fact it was discovered by means of autopsy that some form of coronary atherosclerosis was present in over 77% of the hearts of these soldiers. The extent of this varied from slight "fibrous" thickening to large plaques causing complete occlusion of one or more of the major vessels of the heart.

A person can have atherosclerosis for 50 or 60 years or more and die from some other cause. However, almost 1 million persons in the United States each year are not so fortunate.

Coronary thrombosis

Coronary thrombosis is the medical name for what is commonly referred to by most people as a "heart attack." This occurs when a section of the heart muscle is deprived of its blood supply. The stage is set for the heart attack by the gradual narrowing of the coronary arteries. Most heart attacks are caused when a blood clot, or thrombus, lodges in one of the narrowed coronary arteries—thus limiting the blood supply to a certain area of the heart. Although such an attack may be sudden, it usually is the result of the slowly developing process of atherosclerosis in the coronary arteries.

The symptoms of a heart attack vary from person to person, but the usual symptoms are as follows:

1. Uncomfortable pressure, fullness, and painful sensation in center of chest, lasting for 2 minutes or more.
2. Pain may spread to the shoulders, neck, or arms.
3. Sweating, dizziness, shortness of breath, and nausea may also occur.

It should be noted that sharp, short twinges of pain are not usually signals of a heart attack.

When part of the heart is deprived of sufficient oxygen, certain damage may occur. This damage is referred to as *myocardial infarction*. *Myocardium* is the Latin name of the heart muscle. The word *infarction* simply means death of tissue by loss of its normal supply of oxygenated blood. Thus the term *myocardial infarction* indicates that a small portion of the heart muscle has died because an artery or branch of an artery that formerly supplied it with oxygenated blood has been closed.[18]

Stroke

A stroke occurs when a part of the brain is deprived of its blood supply and as a result the nerve cells in that part of the brain cannot function properly. When this happens, the part of the body controlled by these nerve cells cannot function either.[10]

The importance of a regular supply of oxygen to the brain is clearly demonstrated during prolonged vigorous exercise, when the body demands additional oxygen for use by the working muscles. Blood is diverted from various parts of the body to the working musculature. The brain is the only area to which the blood supply does not change, which demonstrates the importance of a steady supply of blood to the brain. The blood supply to the brain may be impaired by clotting, compression, or hemorrhage.[31]

The most common cause of a stroke is a thrombus becoming lodged in one of the arteries leading to the brain. If this occurs, the blood supply to part of the brain is impaired, and the subject has suffered from what is known as cerebral thrombosis. Again, in the case of a stroke, atherosclerosis is an important underlying cause. A stroke also can be caused by a brain tumor or from excess pressure being placed on the brain or on an artery supplying blood to the brain. A third cause of stroke is bleeding or hemorrhage in an artery supplying blood to the brain. This reduces the supply of blood available to the brain.

Angina pectoris

Angina pectoris is the name given to a chest pain that usually is caused by insufficient blood reaching the heart muscle at times when it is needed. Usually when the demands of the heart cannot be met, it is because of coronary atherosclerosis—the small coronary arteries have become narrowed. Angina pectoris attacks may follow periods of physical exertion or emotional stress. They usually are felt below the sternum, and relief may be obtained by immediate rest.

IDENTIFICATION OF RISK FACTORS

During the past 30 years, attempts have been made to determine the basic cause or causes of heart disease. Large populations have been observed over long periods of time and their living habits and medical records carefully analyzed in relation to the incidence of coronary heart disease. As a result of these studies several factors have been identified which, when present, are associated with an increased risk of cardiovascular disease.

Risk factors that cannot be changed

Four of the risk factors associated with cardiovascular disease cannot be altered by the individual:[19]

1. *Heredity*—Evidence supports the hypothesis that a history of heart disease in the immediate family increases the possibility of cardiovascular illness.
2. *Sex*—Research indicates that the incidence of heart attacks is lower in women under 45 years of age than in men of a comparable age.
3. *Race*—Hypertension, accompanied by a higher incidence of heart attack deaths and stroke, is much more prevalent among black Americans than among whites.
4. *Age*—The incidence of heart attacks and the death rates attributable to them increase with age. For example, for those who are 65 years of age and older, 60% of all deaths are due to cardiovascular disease. This figure is only 11% for those aged 15-24 and 27% for the age group 35-44.

Risk factors that can be altered

Fortunately, the majority of the risk factors can be altered by an adjustment in living habits. These factors include cigarette smoking, high blood pressure, increased levels of cholesterol, obesity, stress, and lack of physical activity.[19]

Cigarette smoking. It is estimated that cigarette smoking is responsible for 325,000 premature deaths each year, with the mortality rate twice as high among cigarette smokers than among nonsmokers.[26] Of this excess mortality, 19% is caused by lung cancer and as much as 37% by coronary heart disease.[5] The following represents a summary of the research available concerning cigarette smoking and cardiovascular disease:

1. Those who smoke cigarettes regularly have a much higher incidence of cardiovascular disease than those who do not smoke.
2. Those with a history of regular cigarette smoking have a considerably higher death

rate from cardiovascular disease than those who do not smoke.

3. The greater the number of cigarettes smoked daily the higher the incidence of coronary disease and the higher the incidence of sudden death following heart disease.

4. Those who stop smoking quickly lower their risk factor of cardiovascular disease to the level of those who do not smoke.

A summary of four studies relating to cigarette smoking is presented in Fig. 2-8. The effect of cigarette smoking on cardiovascular disease is independent of other major factors. However, when other risk factors are present the risk is greatly increased.[30]

High blood pressure. In 1977 the blood pressure of more than 34 million Americans was consistently above the normal range. This condition is referred to as hypertension. It has been demonstrated that an increased blood pressure level accelerates the process of atherosclerosis, with a corresponding increase in cardiovascular disease.

Hypertension may be controlled through medication, diet and weight control, and possibly regular exercise. The role of regular exercise is unclear, but it appears that for those with hypertension, a significant reduction in blood pressure follows a regular cardiovascular exercise program.

Increased levels of cholesterol, triglycerides, and low density lipoproteins. Cholesterol is a member of the lipid or fat family and is essential to the functioning of the body. Some cholesterol is, in fact, manufactured by the body, with normal adults producing approximately 200 mg of this essential fat daily. There are, however, large quantities of cholesterol in certain foods.

Fig. 2-8. Summary of results of four studies relating cigarette smoking and cardiovascular disease.

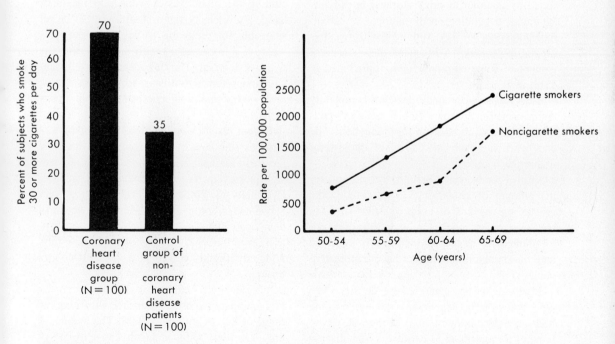

Fig. 2-8, cont'd. Summary of results of four studies relating cigarette smoking and cardiovascular disease.

Table 2-2. Cholesterol content of selected foods

Food	Approximate weight of serving (ounces)	Milligrams cholesterol per serving	Food	Approximate weight of serving (ounces)	Milligrams cholesterol per serving
Beef	3	63	Shrimp	2	76
Pork	3	63	Lobster	2	120
Lamb	3	63	Oysters	2	120
Veal	3	81	Liver	2	180
Fish	3	63	Egg (whole)	1½	275
Chicken	3	54	Tuna	3½	60
Cottage cheese	2	10	Turkey	3	60
Crab	2	76	Margarine	3	65

Foods that are rich in natural cholesterol are the dangerous ones. These usually are referred to as saturated fats. Fats are made up of carbon and hydrogen molecules. If each carbon molecule is combined with two hydrogen molecules, the combination is referred to as a saturated fat. When there are fewer than two hydrogen molecules for each carbon molecule, they are referred to as either monounsaturated or polyunsaturated, depending on the number of carbon molecules that are not combined with two hydrogen molecules.[3] A listing of the cholesterol content of some common foods is included in Table 2-2.

Unfortunately, the body does not completely compensate for this extra dietary supply of cholesterol by cutting back on its production. The end result is an elevated level of cholesterol within the body.

Until recently it was thought that the greater the amount of cholesterol in the blood, the greater the danger of cardiovascular disease. However, recent research now indicates that not all cholesterol in the bloodstream is injurious and that one kind may in fact have a protective value.[4,15,16]

Lipoproteins are classified by density. The type thought to be beneficial is contained in the high density lipoproteins, while the type thought to contribute to cardiovascular disease is contained in the low density lipoproteins.

At birth approximately half of the total cholesterol in the blood is contained in high density lipoprotein. However, as adulthood is reached the amount of high density lipoprotein decreases and the low density lipoprotein increases.

One theory suggests that low density lipoprotein seems to be involved in transporting cholesterol to, and depositing it in, the tissues, including the blood vessel walls. On the other hand, high density lipoprotein seems to be responsible for removing cholesterol from sites where it is in excess and carrying it back to the liver for disposal. Thus it appears that high density lipoprotein may thwart the atherosclerotic process by removing cholesterol from artery walls.

Recent research has shown that members of families who have enjoyed long lives free from heart disease have very high levels of high density lipoprotein. A study conducted at Stanford University by Wood et al.[35] showed that very active men who run at least 15 miles a week had developed high levels of high density lipoprotein, even though their level of total cholesterol was only slightly less than a matched control group.

The level of cholesterol in this country is high compared to other countries, with a normal range of 220 to 260 mg/100 ml. The average is only 150 mg/100 ml in Japan, but only 5% of the population in the United States have a cholesterol level of less than 160 mg/100 ml. In this

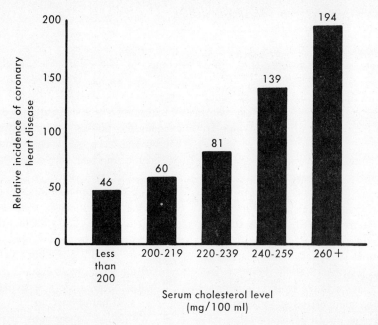

Fig. 2-9. Risk of developing coronary heart disease according to cholesterol levels. (Adapted from Dawber and Kannel.[7])

Fig. 2-10. Serum cholesterol levels in coronary and noncoronary heart disease subjects. (Based on data from Gertler and White.[14])

Fig. 2-11. Effect of a special low-cholesterol diet on the serum cholesterol level. Note that the decrease in the cholesterol level of the special diet group is approximately five times that of the regular diet group. (Based on data from Leren.[24])

country more than 40% of the average diet is derived from fats, whereas in Japan this figure is less than 10%.

The American Heart Association presents three dietary recommendations for those who wish to reduce their chances of cardiovascular disease:

1. A caloric intake adjusted to achieve and maintain the proper weight.
2. A total intake of less than 40% of the total calories from fat, with the ratio of polyunsaturated fat to saturated fat approximately 2:1.
3. A substantial reduction of cholesterol in the diet to less than 300 mg daily.[8]

Research findings relative to this important risk factor can be summarized as follows:

1. A linear relationship exists between the relative incidence of coronary heart disease and the serum cholesterol level: the lower the cholesterol level, the lower the risk of some form of cardiovascular disease; the higher the cholesterol level, the higher the risk of cardiovascular disease (Fig. 2-9).
2. The cholesterol level for subjects who have experienced some form of cardiovascular disease is much higher than for those who have no known associated problems (Fig. 2-10).
3. The average level of cholesterol in the blood can be reduced by as much as 18% if the above recommendations from the American Heart Association are followed (Fig. 2-11).

Obesity and excess weight. The problems of obesity and excess weight have increased to epidemic proportions in the United States during the past 10 to 20 years. In 1966, for example, approximately 35% of the adult population were considered overweight; by 1979, this figure had increased to 62%.[17]

Obesity may be defined as an excess accumulation of body fat over and above what is considered desirable for a person's sex and weight. The average amount of body fat for college-age

men in this country is 15%, while that for women is 25%. Values exceeding these percentages can be considered as approaching obesity.

Excess weight is defined as body weight that exceeds the normal standards based on sex, height, and frame size. The standards that are considered "normal" are usually developed by life insurance companies.

According to Kannel,[22] obesity and/or excess weight has been shown to have a definite relationship to certain cardiovascular diseases, possibly because of the following:

1. Extra stress is placed on the heart because of the added work load.
2. Obesity is closely associated with increased blood pressure.
3. With obesity there is usually an increased level of cholesterol and other lipids.

Thus it would appear advantageous to reduce the amount of body fat or excess body weight in view of the favorable effect this would have on the other related factors. In the Framingham study, subjects who were 20 pounds or more overweight suffered three times as many fatal heart attacks as those who could be considered of normal weight.

High level of emotional stress. Stress is defined as "the physical or emotional factor that causes bodily or mental tension."[33] There are many causal factors determining the level of stress. When these occur, the body is able to overcome the stressor or else there is an increased level of anxiety or tension created within the body. Selye[29] indicates that when an organism is exposed to a stressor, the response is in the form of a general reaction that includes three phases: (1) an alarm reaction, (2) a stage of resistance, and (3) a stage of exhaustion. He further indicates that in some instances the body can prepare for future stress by gradual adaptation to a stressor in small doses.

Much stress may be caused by an individual's occupation. This is referred to as occupation-related stress and is probably the most significant type. Friedman and Rosenman[13] have developed a set of criteria for evaluating a person's stress level. They indicate that a person can be classified into one of two groups. The first of these groups is referred to as type A, which consists of individuals exhibiting a high stress level and rating high on the following criteria:

1. *Ambition*—An intense, sustained drive to achieve self-selected but usually poorly defined goals.
2. *Competitiveness*—A profound inclination and an eagerness to compete.
3. *Aggressiveness*—Persistent desire for recognition and advancement.
4. *Profound sense of time urgency*—Continuous involvement in multiple functions while constantly subject to restrictions.
5. *Drive*—Persistent efforts to accelerate the rate of execution of many physical and mental functions.

These traits are normally present in most individuals, but in the type A person they are present to an excessive degree. Individuals who fall in this group include those who cannot stand to have unscheduled time on their hands and who become very upset when they are kept waiting.

Those who rate low in these traits were classified as type B. This is the type of person who usually is able to relax easily. Very seldom does he let outside factors adversely influence his emotional state. The level of anxiety and tension of a type B person is therefore very low.

In an attempt to determine the relationship between stress level and cardiovascular disease, Friedman and Rosenman[13] compared a group of type A subjects with a group of type B subjects with regard to certain factors relating to heart disease. Each group contained 83 subjects selected so that they did not differ with regard to age, height, weight, total caloric intake, total fat intake, and amount of physical activity. There was a large difference between the two groups with regard to the incidence of coronary heart disease (Fig. 2-12). This was seven times more prevalent in the high stress group than in the low stress group.

The two groups also differed significantly in the amount of cholesterol in the bloodstream (Fig. 2-13). The mean cholesterol level in the

Fig. 2-12. Comparison of Group A (high stress) and Group B (low stress) with regard to incidence of coronary heart disease (age range 30 to 59 years). (Based on data from Friedman and Rosenman.[13])

Fig. 2-13. Comparison of Group A (high stress) and Group B (low stress) with regard to level of serum cholesterol (age range 30 to 59 years). (Based on data from Friedman and Rosenman.[13])

high stress group was 253 mg/100 ml compared to 215 mg/100 ml in the low stress group.

A later study indicated that subjects who were classified as type A experienced difficulty in clearing fat from the bloodstream after ingestion of a high-fat meal.[13] This explains the high cholesterol level found in the subjects.

Later studies by Friedman and Rosenman[13] showed conclusively that the serum cholesterol level is increased when the intensity of type A behavior is increased and is reduced when there is less sense of time urgency. Thus the level of serum cholesterol can be altered by the brain and its functioning.

A summary of information from research relating to this area is as follows:

1. The incidence of coronary heart disease is much higher in those who have a high level of occupational stress.[27]
2. There is a definite, positive relationship between the level of stress and the incidence of cigarette smoking.[27]

Lack of physical activity. In the previous discussion on physical fitness, the sedentary life pattern that exists in this country was emphasized. It was shown that automation, elevators, television sets, and many other mechanical devices have reduced the expenditure of physical effort. With this reduction of physical activity in modern living there has been a concurrent increase not only in the incidence of cardiovascular disease but also in the associated mortality rate.

One cannot prove a causal relationship between the decrease in activity and the increase in cardiovascular disease. There is, however, a growing body of knowledge suggesting that physical inactivity may be one of many possible factors involved in the increasing incidence of coronary heart disease.[11]

The majority of the studies concerning the relationship between regular exercise and other cardiovascular disease risk factors show that regular aerobic exercise will result in the following:

1. A reduction in the level of cholesterol and blood lipids.
2. A reduction in the resting systolic and diastolic blood pressures, particularly if these values are elevated at the start of the training program.
3. A reduction in body weight and/or percentage of body fat.
4. A reduction in the incidence of abnormalities occurring during an exercise electrocardiogram.[1]

These factors would explain, at least in part, why several studies have shown that persons in physically active jobs have a much lower incidence of coronary heart disease than persons in physically inactive jobs.[20,25]

It also has been shown in several studies that the level of activity is closely associated with

Fig. 2-14. Relationship between death associated with coronary heart disease and level of activity. Note the higher incidence in the death rate among the least active group. (Adapted from Frank et al.[12])

the early mortality rate following an initial heart attack. Data obtained by Frank et al.[12] are presented in Fig. 2-14. The mortality rate was found to be almost three times as great in the subjects classified as least active (49%) as that obtained for the most active subjects (17%).

Similar results were obtained by Brunner.[2] He followed carefully for 6 years 282 subjects who experienced an initial heart attack. He found that in the first 4 weeks after the attack 4.2% of the active workers died, whereas 22.6% of the sedentary workers died. After 6 years 23.1% of the active workers had died, whereas 59% of the inactive group had died. (See Fig. 2-15.)

SUMMARY

The circulatory system is a most important system, for all other systems of the body depend on it. As energy is required for the performance of all activity, the efficiency with which the body can circulate the blood is an important factor in the determination of the amount of work that the body can perform. Also, by having a complete knowledge of the construction and function of the circulatory system

it will be possible to understand more fully certain aspects of cardiovascular disease.

Several risk factors associated with a higher incidence of cardiovascular disease have been presented, and evidence from associated research has been discussed. It should be stressed that in no instance can a cause-effect relationship be established between one or all of these factors and the occurrence of a heart attack; however, the evidence does appear to be conclusive that a person can reduce his chances of suffering a heart attack by taking positive action concerning several of these risk factors. As was quoted previously, "If the knowledge we have now were properly applied we could halve the number of deaths from coronary attacks; in short, we could probably save over 200,000 lives a year."[21]

Students can be made aware of ways in which they can reduce their chances of suffering from some form of cardiovascular disease. In the game called RISKO, developed by the Michigan Heart Association, one can estimate his chances of suffering a heart attack. Read the instructions carefully and determine which category you are classified in.

Fig. 2-15. Death rates associated with coronary heart disease, according to activity level. (Adapted from Brunner.[2])

RISKO

The purpose of this game is to give you an estimate of your chances of suffering heart attack.

The game is played by making squares which — from left to right — represent an increase in your RISK FACTORS. These are medical conditions and habits associated with an increased danger of heart attack. *Not all risk factors are measurable enough to be included in this game;*

RULES:

Study each RISK FACTOR AND its row. Find the box applicable to you and circle the large number in it. For example, if you are 37, circle the number in the box labeled 31-40.
After checking out all the rows, add the circled numbers. This total — your score — is an estimate of your risk.

IF YOU SCORE:

6-11 — Risk well below
average
12-17 — Risk below average
18-24 — Risk generally average

25-31 — Risk moderate
32-40 — Risk at a dangerous level
41-62 — Danger urgent. See your
doctor now.

HEREDITY:

Count parents, grand-parents, brothers, and sisters who have had heart attack and/or stroke.

TOBACCO SMOKING:

If you inhale deeply and smoke a cigarette way down, add one to your classification. Do NOT subtract because you think you do not inhale or smoke only a half inch on a cigarette.

EXERCISE:

Lower your score one point if you exercise regularly and frequently.

CHOLESTEROL OR SATURATED FAT INTAKE LEVEL:

A cholesterol blood level is best. If you can't get one from your doctor, then estimate honestly the percentage of solid fats you eat. These are usually of animal origin — lard, cream, butter, and beef and lamb fat. If you eat much of this, your cholesterol level probably will be high. The U.S. average, 40%, is too high for good health.

BLOOD PRESSURE:

If you have no recent reading but have passed an insurance or industrial examination chances are you are 140 or less.

SEX:

This line takes into account the fact that men have from 6 to 10 times more heart attacks than women of child bearing age.

	1	2	3	4	6	8
AGE	10 to 20	21 to 30	31 to 40	41 to 50	51 to 60	61 to 70 and over
HEREDITY	No known history of heart disease	1 relative with cardiovascular disease Over 60	2 relatives with cardiovascular disease Over 60	1 relative with cardiovascular disease Under 60	2 relatives with cardiovascular disease Under 60	3 relatives with cardiovascular disease Under 60
WEIGHT	More than 5 lbs. below standard weight	—5 to +5 lbs. standard weight	6-20 lbs. over weight	21-35 lbs. over weight	36-50 lbs. over weight	51-65 lbs. over weight
TOBACCO SMOKING	Non-user	Cigar and/or pipe	10 cigarettes or less a day	20 cigarettes a day	30 cigarettes a day	40 cigarettes a day or more
EXERCISE	Intensive occupational and recreational exertion	Moderate occupational and recreational exertion	Sedentary work and intense recreational exertion	Sedentary occupational and moderate recreational exertion	Sedentary work and light recreational exertion	Complete lack of all exercise
CHOLESTEROL OR FAT % IN DIET	Cholesterol below 180 mg.% Diet contains no animal or solid fats	Cholesterol 181-205 mg.% Diet contains 10% animal or solid fats	Cholesterol 206-230 mg.% Diet contains 20% animal or solid fats	Cholesterol 231-255 mg.% Diet contains 30% animal or solid fats	Cholesterol 256-280 mg.% Diet contains 40% animal or solid fats	Cholesterol 281-300 mg.% Diet contains 50% animal or solid fats
BLOOD PRESSURE	100 upper reading	120 upper reading	140 upper reading	160 upper reading	180 upper reading	200 or over upper reading
SEX	Female under 40	Female 40-50	Female over 50	Male	Stocky male	Bald stocky male

REFERENCES

1. Blackburn, H., et al.: Premature ventricular complexes induced by stress testing, American Journal of Cardiology, **31**:441, April, 1973.
2. Brunner, D.: The influence of physical activity on incidence and prognosis of ischemic heart disease. In Raab, W., editor: Prevention of ischemic heart disease, Springfield, Ill., 1966, Charles C Thomas, Publisher, p. 236.
3. Cant, G.: What you must know about diet. In The healthy life, New York, 1966, Time, Inc., pp. 64-71.
4. Castelli, W. P.: High blood lipid levels can be good or bad—depending on the lipid, The Journal of the American Medical Association, **237**:1066, 1977.
5. Cigarette smoking and cardiovascular disease, Dallas, 1977, American Heart Association, p. 5.
6. The circulatory system, Public Health Service publication no. 482, Washington, D.C., 1964, U.S. Department of Health, Education and Welfare, p. 16.
7. Dawber, T. R., and Kannel, W. B.: Susceptibility to coronary artery disease, Modern Concepts of Cardiovascular Disease **30**:671-673, July, 1961.
8. Diet and Coronary Heart Disease, Dallas, 1978, American Heart Association, pp. 3-5.
9. Enos, W. F., Holmes, R. H., and Beyer, J.: Coronary disease among United States soldiers killed in action in Korea, The Journal of the American Medical Association **152**:1090, 1953.
10. Facts about strokes, New York, 1964, American Heart Association, p. 2.
11. Fox, S., and Skinner, J.: Physical activity and cardiovascular health, American Journal of Cardiology **14**: 731, Dec., 1964.
12. Frank, C. W., Wainblatt, E., Shapiro, S., et al.: Physical inactivity as a lethal factor in myocardial infarction among men, Circulation **34**:1022, Dec., 1966.
13. Friedman, M., and Rosenman, R. H.: Type A behavior and your heart, Greenwich, Conn., 1975, Fawcett Publications, Inc.
14. Gertler, M. M., and White, P. D.: Coronary heart disease in young adults, Cambridge, Mass., 1954, Commonwealth Fund.
15. Gettman, L. R.: Concerning cholesterol, Aero-Ac'cent, Vol. 8, No. 1, 1980, p. 5.
16. Hartung, G., and Squires, W. G.: Exercise and HDL cholesterol in middle age men, Physician and Sports Medicine, **8**:74, Jan., 1980.
17. Health maintenance, Newport Beach, Calif., Nov., 1978, Pacific Mutual Life Insurance Co.
18. Heart attack, New York, 1956, American Heart Association, p. 3.
19. Heart facts, 1980, Dallas, 1980, American Heart Association, p. 5.
20. Hickey, N., et al.: Study of coronary risk factors related to physical activities in 15,171 men, British Medical Journal **3**:507, 1975.
21. High blood pressure, New York, 1966, American Heart Association, p. 3.
22. Kannel, W. Cited in Berg, R. H.: No more heart attacks, Look, Feb. 2, 1969, p. 30.
23. Kannel, W.: Habits and coronary heart disease. The Framingham heart study, Public Health Service publication no. 1515, Bethesda, Md., 1968, U.S. Department of Health, Education and Welfare, p. 4.
24. Leren, P.: The effect of plasma cholesterol lowering diet in male survivors of myocardial infarction, Acta Medica Scandinavica **466**(supp.):1, 1966.
25. Paffenbarger, R. S., and Hale, W. E.: Work activities and coronary heart mortality, The New England Journal of Medicine **292**:545, 1975.
26. Proceedings of Third World Conference on Smoking and Health, 1975: Vol. I, Modifying the risk for the smoker, Washington, D.C., U.S. Department of Health, Education and Welfare.
27. Russek, H. I.: Emotional stress, tobacco smoking, and ischemic heart disease. In Raab, W., editor: Prevention of ischemic heart disease, Springfield, Ill., 1966, Charles C Thomas, Publisher, p. 190.
28. Sanders, H. J.: Heart disease. In Jones, H. L., editor: Science and theory of health, Dubuque, Iowa, 1966, Wm. C. Brown Company, Publishers, p. 235.
29. Selye, H.: The stress of life, New York, 1956, Blakiston Division, McGraw-Hill Book Co., Inc.
30. Shurtleff, D.: Some characteristics related to the incidence of cardiovascular diseases and death: Framingham study, eighteen years follow-up, Washington, D.C., U.S. Department of Health, Education and Welfare, 1974.
31. Strokes—agenda for the family, New York, 1958, American Heart Association, pp. 5-8.
32. Varicose veins, New York, 1961, American Heart Association, p. 5.
33. Webster's seventh new collegiate dictionary, Springfield, Mass., 1965, G. & C. Merriam Company, p. 868.
34. The wonderful human machine, Chicago, 1961, American Medical Association, p. 26.
35. Wood, P. D., et al.: Distribution of plasma lipoproteins in middle-age male runners, Metabolism, **25**:1249, Nov., 1976.

CHAPTER 3

Physical fitness

What do you know about physical fitness?

T F

☐ ☐ **1.** The increased emphasis on physical fitness during the past 20 years has resulted in a significant improvement in the physical fitness level in this country.

☐ ☐ **2.** There is an increased need for people to participate in organized physical activity.

☐ ☐ **3.** The incidence of cardiovascular disease is higher in this country than in any other country.

☐ ☐ **4.** A large number of people in this country believe that they should exercise more. Most people who do not exercise regularly lack sufficient time to do so.

☐ ☐ **5.** Most people in this country exhibit an adequate level of physical fitness.

☐ ☐ **6.** The minimal level of physical fitness will be the same for everyone.

☐ ☐ **7.** Attaining a maximal level of physical fitness should be a goal for most college students.

☐ ☐ **8.** Only factors that relate to the development of health and increase the functional capacity of the body should be classified as physical fitness components.

☐ ☐ **9.** The four components of physical fitness are strength, endurance, flexibility, and speed.

☐ ☐ **10.** Physical fitness is defined as the ability to perform sports skills correctly.

There is a recognized desire in the United States to improve the physical fitness level of children and adults. The problem was first called to public attention in 1955 by President Dwight D. Eisenhower when he turned his attention to the vital problem of physical fitness. As a former general of the army, he was aware of the inadequate fitness level of young men reporting for military service. Studies made after World War II indicate that nearly 50% of all draft age men had to be rejected or given noncombat jobs because of physical inadequacies.[9]

He also treated with respect and concern the report by Kraus and Hirschland,[6] which indicated that the youth of the United States were inferior to European youth in the performance of six selected tests designed to measure minimal muscular fitness. The results, presented in Fig. 3-1, indicate that in European countries only 8% failed one or more of these tests, whereas 57% failed in the United States. These tests were designed to measure only *minimal* levels of muscular fitness.

As a result, the President's Council on Physical Fitness was established, and following President Eisenhower's example, both President John F. Kennedy and President Lyndon B. Johnson exhibited an extreme interest in the improvement of the physical fitness level of adults and children in this country. President Johnson emphasized that "physical fitness is a matter of fundamental importance to individual well-being and to the progress and security of our nation."[11] President Kennedy referred to physical fitness as "the basis of all other forms of excellence."

In a 1980 address President Jimmy Carter indicated that regular participation in a good physical fitness program is the best possible investment in American health. "Everything we do to make Americans more physically fit," he said, "pays off handsomely. It cuts medical bills, it helps our people to live longer, and it adds to the quality of each day of life that we live."[8]

Many prominent persons in the field of medicine and in other fields have spoken and written about the need for exercise in maintaining an organically sound body from birth through old age. Governors and legislators have called conferences to motivate the people of their states to begin physical fitness programs.

One might ask why the sudden emphasis on physical fitness. One reason is that the tasks of daily life no longer provide sufficient vigorous exercise to develop and maintain "adequate" levels of physical fitness. With increased mechanization there has been a corresponding

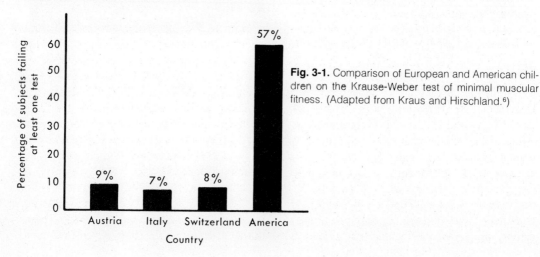

Fig. 3-1. Comparison of European and American children on the Krause-Weber test of minimal muscular fitness. (Adapted from Kraus and Hirschland.[6])

decrease in the number of tasks that require an expenditure of energy.

The sedentary way of life has had a negative effect on the human body and has been associated with many health problems. Pollock et al.[12] state that "serious medical problems such as coronary heart disease, hypertension, obesity, anxiety and depression, and lower back pain problems have been either directly or indirectly related to lack of physical activity." These diseases and conditions have been referred to by Kraus and Raab as hypokinetic diseases, or diseases associated with insufficient physical activity.

Recent statistics for this country concerning physical fitness and health were presented in Chapter 1. These statistics indicate that most Americans have unhealthy habits and live unhealthy lives. One of the problems associated with changing these habits is that Americans' life-styles have little effect on their health *now*. The absence of any immediate effect is a serious barrier to change. As long as individuals feel well, they often will think they are physically fit and will not want to initiate a change in their life-styles.

It is interesting to note that less than 20% of the American adult population rated their own level of health less than adequate. This figure was not very much higher among those who are overweight, who smoke, and who do not exercise regularly.[4]

It would appear that the maintenance of an adequate level of physical fitness is essential for anyone wishing to make the most of himself and of his life, and that many advantages result from achieving and maintaining an adequate level of physical fitness. Most Americans are aware of the benefits that can be derived from regular exercise, and many of them intend to exercise more, but for some reason or another they just do not get around to doing this. If a person believes strongly enough in exercise, he will make time available to participate in an activity program on a regular basis. Unfortu-

nately, too few Americans believe strongly enough to do this.

DEFINITION OF PHYSICAL FITNESS

Despite the widespread interest in physical fitness, it is still difficult to define it in a manner that is acceptable to all concerned. The American Association for Health, Physical Education, Recreation, and Dance defines fitness as follows:

Fitness is that state which characterizes the degree to which a person is able to function efficiently. Fitness is an individual matter. It implies the ability of each person to live most effectively within his potentialities. Ability to function depends upon the physical, mental, emotional, social, moral, and spiritual components of fitness, all of which are related to each other and are mutually interdependent.[2]

Clarke defines physical fitness as "the ability to carry out daily tasks with vigor and alertness, without undue fatigue, and with ample energy to enjoy leisure time pursuits and to meet unforeseen emergencies."[1] He further indicates that "physical fitness is the ability to last, to bear up and to persevere under difficult circumstances where an unfit person would give up. It is the opposite to being fatigued from ordinary efforts, to lacking the energy to enter zestfully into life's activities, and to becoming exhausted from unexpected, demanding physical exertion."[3]

Physical fitness is an individual matter and as such has little meaning unless viewed in relation to the specific needs of each individual. The minimal level that is necessary will vary according to the needs of each individual, who must decide for himself whether or not this is sufficient. It is rather unfortunate that many individuals do not realize just how high a level of physical fitness is actually necessary. Many persons when asked if they participate regularly in an exercise program indicate that this is not necessary because their level of physical fitness is adequate for their everyday tasks. These, however, are often the same persons who complain of several of the symptoms that are listed in Table 3-1. If several of these symptoms are applicable to you, it is doubtful that you have an adequate level of physical fitness.

As was indicated previously, physical fitness is an individual matter. The amount of activity required by each individual in performing everyday tasks will determine the kind and degree of physical fitness that is necessary. It has been suggested that physical fitness should be considered as a continuum, or scale, ranging from very low levels to maximum levels (Fig. 3-2). Each person has some degree of physical

Table 3-1. Symptoms associated with less than adequate standards of physical fitness*

Symptom	Check if applicable to you
1. Yawning at your desk	☐
2. Drowsy feeling all day	☐
3. Prone to temper tantrums	☐
4. Fatigue from minimal exertion	☐
5. Too tired to pursue leisure activities	☐
6. Nervous, jittery condition	☐
7. Difficult to relax	☐
8. Subject to worries and moods	☐
9. Irritable disposition toward others	☐

*Based on data from Cooper, K. H.: Aerobics, New York, 1968, M. Evans and Company.

fitness and would thus fit somewhere on this continuum. An individual who is able to meet the demands of each day only with difficulty and who suffers from fatigue and lack of energy would be placed toward the lower end of this scale. According to Johnson et al.:

> The subminimal level of physical fitness is characterized by physical inefficiency and quite often by some degree of emotional instability. He is easily "fatigued," often "edgy" and unable to meet physical or emotional challenges head on with confidence, determination and a reasonable share of success.[5]

It is also possible to consider additional degrees of physical fitness. A person who is able to meet the demands of the day without difficulty and with relative ease would be higher on the scale, toward the maximal level. Somewhere along this scale is a point representing an adequate level of physical fitness, This has been defined as the ability to meet the demands of life with vigor and alertness, without undue fatigue, and to have sufficient energy beyond this to enjoy leisure time activities and meet unexpected emergencies.

There are many points on this scale ranging up to what could be classified as maximal physical fitness. This is a theoretical point, for although it is never actually determined, we know that there is a maximal level for each individual. The highly trained marathon runner, or any highly trained athlete, could be considered as approaching this point. This level, however, is not a required objective for each individual. Each person is fit when his capacities are devel-

Low	Adequate	Maximal
Low (able to meet the demands only with difficulty— suffers from fatigue and lack of energy)	Adequate (able to meet the demands without undue fatigue—has a reserve of energy)	

Fig. 3-2. Physical fitness continuum. Each person fits somewhere on this continuum, based on his level of physical fitness. The higher his level of physical fitness, the further he will be toward the maximal level. (Adapted from Johnson, Updyke, Stolberg, and Schafer.[5])

oped and maintained at a level near his individual capacity for the demands that are most likely to be made on him in the future.[10]

A person can change his position on this scale. If he neglects the needs of the body for physical activity, it will probably result in a shift to the left. A well-designed exercise program that is followed regularly will, in all probability, result in a shift to the right. It is hoped that more people will realize that a minimal physical fitness level may not be sufficient for the ability to meet the demands of tomorrow.[10] An additional level of physical fitness affords the individual an added margin of safety. A greater supply of energy will result in freedom from fatigue and will possibly increase the enjoyment of daily living.

PRESENT STATUS OF PHYSICAL FITNESS IN THIS COUNTRY

Despite the widespread interest in physical fitness during the past 10 years, American boys and girls did not improve their level of physical fitness. Girls have improved slightly in a small number of tests; however, the average fitness scores recorded in 1975 are almost exactly identical to the scores recorded 10 years earlier.[7]

In a 1980 address[8] President Carter indicated that improving the fitness of children and youth is our biggest challenge and opportunity. He noted that the scores on the National Youth Fitness Test have not improved in 15 years and suggested that American youth have not become fully involved in the fitness movement that is beginning to sweep the country.

PHYSICAL FITNESS COMPONENTS

There has been much confusion in the past concerning the components of physical fitness. Several factors associated with skillful performance of an activity have erroneously been referred to as physical fitness components.

In an effort to clarify this situation, the American Association for Health, Physical Education, Recreation, and Dance has recently adopted a new approach.[2] Physical fitness has now been dichotomized into two areas: health-related physical fitness and performance-related physical fitness.

Health-related fitness refers to those factors that relate to the development of health and increase the functional capacity of the body. The basic components of health-related fitness are cardiovascular endurance, strength, muscular endurance, flexibility, and body composition. Each will be discussed in detail in the following chapters. Methods and programs for improving each of these will be presented along with practical tests that can be used to evaluate the present level of fitness of each person for each of these components. It is well documented that these factors offer the individual some protection against such degenerative diseases as coronary heart disease, obesity, low back pain, hypertension, and various musculoskeletal disorders. This type of fitness should be of primary concern to each individual within our society and should be emphasized because of the improved health benefits that possibly result from regular participation in a good exercise program.

Performance-related fitness includes those factors that are critical to skillful performance in various physical activities. Factors such as speed, reaction time, agility, power, balance, and coordination are of the utmost importance when skill is considered. In the past this area has been referred to as motor ability and will be discussed in detail in Chapter 10.

REFERENCES

1. Clarke, H. H.: Application of measurement to health and physical education, ed. 5, Englewood Cliffs, N.J., 1976, Prentice-Hall, Inc. p. 18.
2. Falls, H. B.: Modern concepts of physical fitness, Journal of Health, Physical Education, and Recreation, **51:**25, April, 1980.
3. From Fitness for Youth, Journal of Health, Physical Education, and Recreation **39:**48, Sept., 1968.
4. Health maintenance, Newport Beach, Calif., 1978, Pacific Mutual Life Insurance Co.

5. Johnson, P. B., Updyke, W. F., Stolberg, D. C., and Schafer, M.: Physical education: a problem-solving approach to health and fitness, New York, 1966, Holt, Rinehart and Winston, Inc., p. 16.

6. Kraus, H., and Hirschland, R.: Physical fitness for children, Research Quarterly **25:**178, May, 1954.

7. Newsletter, April, 1976, President's Council on Physical Fitness and Sports, p. 4.

8. Newsletter, March, 1980, President's Council on Physical Fitness and Sports, p. 2.

9. Olson, E. C.: Conditioning fundamentals, Columbus, Ohio, 1968, Charles E. Merrill Publishing Company, p. 1.

10. Peebler, J. R.: Controlled exercise for physical fitness, Springfield, Ill., 1962, Charles C Thomas, Publisher, p. 4.

11. Physical fitness facts, Washington, D.C., 1968, U.S. Government Printing Office, p. 1.

12. Pollock, M., Wilmore, J., and Fox, S., III: Health and fitness through physical activity, New York, 1978, John Wiley and Sons, Inc., p. 3.

CHAPTER **4**

Cardiovascular endurance

What do you know about cardiovascular endurance?

T F

☐ ☐ **1.** Cardiovascular endurance is the most important component of physical fitness.

☐ ☐ **2.** Endurance is not very important for people who have desk jobs because they do not require very much energy.

☐ ☐ **3.** The main contributing factor to physical work capacity is the strength of the skeletal muscles.

☐ ☐ **4.** The amount of work an individual can perform is largely dependent on the amount of oxygen the body is capable of processing.

☐ ☐ **5.** The body can store an adequate supply of oxygen.

☐ ☐ **6.** An aerobic task is usually a task that is so vigorous it can be maintained for only a short period of time.

☐ ☐ **7.** A very short task of high intensity is largely dependent on the supply of energy anaerobically.

☐ ☐ **8.** An activity must produce a maximal heart rate if it is to contribute to the development of cardiovascular endurance.

☐ ☐ **9.** Maximal oxygen intake can be predicted accurately from the results of the 12-minute-run tests.

☐ ☐ **10.** Chinning the bar 10 to 12 times daily is one of the best methods for development of cardiovascular endurance.

☐ ☐ **11.** Because of the high level of muscular strength a weight lifter possesses, he will also have a high degree of cardiovascular endurance.

☐ ☐ **12.** The 5-minute step test is just as good as the 12-minute run test for predicting aerobic capacity.

Because more than 55% of all deaths in the United States are attributable to cardiovascular disease, we should have deep concern for the development of the cardiovascular system. Cardiovascular endurance may be defined as the ability to continue or persist in strenuous tasks involving large muscle groups for long periods of time. In more simple terms it may be defined as the maximal amount of work that an individual can perform over an extended period of time. Large muscle groups should be involved in the work tasks, which should be fairly simple so that the mechanical efficiency is kept relatively constant.

The capacity for heavy prolonged muscular work depends on the body's ability to supply oxygen to the working muscles. The more oxygen the body is able to take in and utilize, the more work the body should be capable of producing. The heart and circulatory and respiratory systems must function efficiently if a high degree of cardiovascular endurance is to be achieved. In recent years this is the one component of physical fitness that has been stressed because of the various health advantages associated with the development of high levels of cardiovascular endurance. It is difficult to determine what advantages are associated with a high level of strength or flexibility, and it has been emphasized that a minimal level of these is adequate for most individuals. However, there are certain benefits that can be derived from attaining above average levels of cardiovascular endurance. These will be discussed in detail in the chapter devoted to exercise and health.

MAXIMAL OXYGEN INTAKE

Just as there is a maximal heart rate that can be attained during exercise, so there is a maximal amount of oxygen the body is able to use. This is referred to as the maximal oxygen intake or aerobic capacity. This measure is recognized by most authorities to be the best measure of a person's cardiovascular fitness.

The amount of oxygen that can be processed by the body is dependent on the following:

1. *Adequate ventilation.* Air must be moved in and out of the lungs.
2. *Amount of hemoglobin.* This will determine the amount of oxygen that can be carried by the blood.
3. *Cardiac output.* The more blood circulated, the more oxygen that will be available.
4. *Amount of oxygen extracted from the blood.* The ability of the cells to use the oxygen circulated will determine the maximal amount of oxygen that can be used by the body.

The relationship between oxygen consumption and energy expenditure can be summarized as follows:

1. *Each activity requires energy.* Every activity that must be performed by the body requires energy. Even simple activities such as sitting and sleeping require a certain amount of energy.
2. *To produce energy, oxygen is necessary.* Energy is produced by the burning of foodstuffs, but oxygen is the necessary burning agent.
3. *The body can store food, but it cannot store oxygen.* It is necessary for a person to breathe in order to live. If the oxygen supply is discontinued, the body quickly dies, since the oxygen supply in the body will last for only a limited period of time.

When the demands for oxygen increase within the body, as in strenuous exercise, the ability of the body to take in and deliver oxygen to the working musculature will be an important factor in determining how much work can be performed. The more oxygen the circulatory and respiratory systems are able to deliver, the longer the person will be able to exercise before fatigue or exhaustion sets in. As an individual continues running, his performance will deteriorate after a period of time as it becomes difficult for him to continue. The reason is that each person reaches the point at which his body cannot process sufficient oxygen to supply the energy needed to perform the task. Cooper indicates the following when this point is reached:

. . . each of you should look at what your body is doing in its noble effort to keep you going. Your

Fig. 4-1. Relative roles of anaerobic and aerobic oxidation for supplying total amounts of oxygen.

chest is heaving as the lungs try to bring in more oxygen. Your heart is pounding as it tries to pump more blood which carries the oxygen around your body. The blood is racing through the blood vessels to every extremity as it tries to deliver more oxygen. It's the condition of these systems and others which determines your cardiovascular fitness and it's the improvement of these systems toward which all exercise should be directed.[2]

Aerobic-anaerobic work

The total amount of work of which an individual is capable may be determined by the amount of aerobic work that can be performed, the amount of anaerobic work that can be performed, or a combination of both.

Aerobic work may be defined as work in which the amount of oxygen taken in and used by the body is sufficient to provide the energy necessary for the performance of the task.

Anaerobic work is work in which the amount of oxygen that the body can supply is less than the amount necessary to perform the task. Anaerobic work can be performed *only* for short periods of time, since an "oxygen debt" is incurred, and there is a buildup of lactic acid in the bloodstream.

Balke[1] clearly demonstrates the role of the oxygen debt capacity for the performance of exercises requiring nearly all-out effort for time intervals from 1 to 15 minutes. That a very short effort is accomplished almost entirely anaerobically can readily be seen. The relation-

ship between the two is clearly demonstrated in Fig. 4-1. This graph indicates that during a 1-minute run approximately 60% of the work is performed anaerobically. During a 4-minute run this decreases to approximately 20%, and during an 8-minute task only approximately 10% of the energy is still supplied anaerobically. It can be seen that for work periods exceeding 10 minutes the anaerobic phase becomes less important for the performance of the total work and actually accounts for not more than 5% of the total required amounts of oxygen. Thus any task continued for 10 minutes or more gives an adequate estimate of the individual's aerobic capacity if he performs the maximal amount of work during this time period.

DEVELOPMENT OF CARDIOVASCULAR ENDURANCE

Cooper[2] has indicated that if an activity is to contribute to the development of cardiovascular endurance, it must produce a heart rate in excess of 150 beats per minute and that such improvement begins only after this rate of activity has been sustained for at least 5 minutes. These findings are in agreement with an earlier study by Karvonen.[5] Working with untrained subjects he found that if an activity was to improve the exercise tolerance of the heart, it must produce a heart rate in excess of the value located 60% of the way between the resting and the maximal heart rates. For most untrained subjects this critical threshold value was between 140 and 150 beats per minute. To learn which activities are most stressful to the heart and can be used when an overload is necessary for the development of cardiovascular endurance is important. Identifying activities that are less stressful also is important. This information allows the individual to increase the efficiency of his heart by overloading it at times and allowing it to slow down at other times. Activities that satisfy these criteria are considered good activities for the development of cardiovascular endurance. They are usually the continuous activities such as running, swimming, bicycling, basketball, and handball.

A more complete description of the effects of various activities will be presented in Chapter 12.

MEASUREMENT OF CARDIOVASCULAR ENDURANCE

The measurement of maximal oxygen intake is the best measure of an individual's cardiovascular endurance. However, this is not a practical test to administer in terms of either time or equipment, since it involves much time and expensive equipment to administer this test in a controlled laboratory setting.

A reliable estimate of the maximal oxygen consumption may be obtained from the performance during the 12-minute run test. The results of this test correlate very highly (r = +.90) with maximal oxygen intake, and this test is therefore adequate to predict a person's maximal oxygen intake.[3,4]

12-minute run test

Description of test. During a 12-minute period, each person attempts to run as far as possible and should try to maintain a steady pace throughout. An attempt should be made to increase this speed during the latter part of the performance. The number of laps completed during this time will be counted and recorded, and the actual distance covered in this time period will be calculated.

Results from research clearly show close agreement between the objective criterion of maximal oxygen intake actually obtained in a laboratory situation using the necessary equipment and the estimated values obtained from the results of this field test. One can clearly see that the duration of the running test must be between 10 and 20 minutes to predict the maximal oxygen intake reliably.

Results. The results should be recorded in the spaces provided for them.

Number of laps completed _____

Distance of 1 lap _____ feet

Distance covered = Laps × Distance of 1 lap

= _____ × _____

= _____ feet

To convert to miles, divide by 5,280

Distance covered = Distance covered in feet/5,280

= _____/5,280

= _____ miles

(calculate this to 2 decimal places)

Interpretation. The results of this 12-minute field test should be interpreted according to Table 4-1.

Table 4-1. Classification of scores obtained for 12-minute field test

Fitness category	Men (distance covered)	Women (distance covered)
Very poor	Less than 1.19 miles	Less than 1.01 miles
Poor	1.20-1.23 miles	1.02-1.19 miles
Average	1.24-1.53 miles	1.20-1.27 miles
Good	1.54-1.84 miles	1.28-1.42 miles
Excellent	More than 1.84 miles	More than 1.42 miles

1½-mile run test

The 1½-mile run test may be preferred to the 12-minute run test because of the advantage of the ease of administration. The aim of the test is to cover 1½ miles in the shortest time possible. Elapsed time is recorded in minutes and seconds. The results of the 1½-mile run test should be interpreted according to Table 4-2.

Step test

Many different versions of the step test are available for use. Probably the most commonly used is the original 5-minute step test. This test and other variations of it are not as good as the 12-minute run test, but because of practical considerations it is used frequently in the teaching situation.

An accurate measurement of the heart rate is necessary if the results of this test are to be meaningful. Heart rate may be counted most easily by pressing gently with the fingertips on the radial artery that is located on the lateral side of the wrist or on one of the carotid arteries that pass anteriorly in the neck. The place where the pulse can be detected most easily should be used. For the purpose of this evaluation, the pulse will be counted for ½-minute periods and then converted to beats per minute by multiplying the obtained value by 2. Each student will practice counting his heart rate by taking four ½-minute counts while remaining seated. Students should refrain from talking and unnecessary movement during periods when heart rates are being counted, since these activities can influence the results obtained. Results should be recorded in Table 4-3.

The step test is based on the premise that for a given submaximal work task the person with a higher level of cardiovascular fitness not only will have a smaller increase in heart rate, but also following the task the heart rate will return to normal much faster than a person's who has a lower level of cardiovascular endurance.

Purpose. The purpose of this test is to obtain immediate knowledge of the level of cardiovascular efficiency.

Table 4-2. Classification of scores obtained for the 1½ mile run test

Classification	Men (time for 1½ miles)	Women (time for 1½ miles)
Very poor	More than 15 min	More than 17.30 min
Poor	14.30-14.59	15.15-17.29
Average	11.45-14.29	14.15-15.14
Good	9.45-11.44	12.45-14.14
Excellent	9.44 or less	12.44 or less

Table 4-3. Heart rate reliability

Trial	Beats per ½ minute		Beats per minute
1	_____	× 2 =	_____
2	_____	× 2 =	_____
3	_____	× 2 =	_____
4	_____	× 2 =	_____

Method. Students should not perform any type of activity prior to this test, and no warm-up should be allowed. A 20-inch bench should be used for men, whereas a 16-inch bench is recommended for women. Each subject steps up to and down from this bench at the rate of 30 steps per minute. The same foot must start the "step-up" each time, and an erect posture must be assumed. The subject continues the activity for a maximum of 5 minutes or, if unable to continue for 5 minutes, he continues until he is no longer able to maintain the set rate. The heart rate is determined for a ½-minute period, starting exactly 1 minute after completion of the last step, that is, from 1 to 1½ minutes after completion of the task.

Results. The results should be recorded in the spaces provided for them.

Table 4-4. Scoring for the Harvard step test*

Duration of effort (min)	TOTAL HEART BEATS 1 TO 1½ MINUTES IN RECOVERY (SCORE—ARBITRARY UNITS)											
	40-44	45-49	50-54	55-59	60-64	65-69	70-74	75-79	80-84	85-89	90-94	95-99
0-½	6	6	5	5	4	4	4	4	3	3	3	3
½-1	19	17	16	14	13	12	11	11	10	9	9	8
1-1½	32	29	26	24	22	20	19	18	17	16	15	14
1½-2	45	41	38	34	31	29	27	25	23	22	21	20
2-2½	58	52	47	43	40	36	34	32	30	28	27	25
2½-3	71	64	58	53	48	45	42	39	37	34	33	31
3-3½	84	75	68	62	57	53	49	46	43	41	39	37
3½-4	97	87	79	72	66	61	57	53	50	47	45	42
4-4½	110	98	89	82	75	70	65	61	57	54	51	48
4½-5	123	110	100	91	84	77	72	68	63	60	57	54
5	129	116	105	96	88	82	76	71	67	63	60	56

INSTRUCTIONS FOR USING THIS TABLE

1. Find the appropriate line for the time stepping was continued.
2. Find the appropriate column for the pulse count for the 30-second period; do *not* multiply this by 2—it is a 30-second count that is used.
3. Read off the score where this line and column intersect.

*From Consolazio, F., Johnson, R., and Pecora, L.: Physiological measurement of metabolic functions in man. Copyright 1963 and used with permission of McGraw-Hill Book Co.

Table 4-5. Classification of Harvard step test scores*

Score	Cardiovascular classification
Below 55	Very poor
56-64	Poor
65-79	Average
80-89	Good
90 or above	Excellent

*If the lowest row of bleachers is used and these are only 16 inches high, a separate set of standards is presented in the cardiovascular profile chart for men on p. 44.

Time of stepping _____ seconds

Heart rate _____ beats per ½ minute

(1 to 1½ minutes of recovery)

The physical efficiency index (PEI) may be calculated or it may be easily estimated by consulting Table 4-4.

The procedure for calculating the PEI is as follows:

$$PEI = \frac{\text{Time of stepping in seconds} \times 100}{5.5 \times \text{Heart rate for ½ minute}}$$

$$= \frac{\underline{\hspace{3cm}} \times 100}{5.5 \times \underline{\hspace{2cm}}}$$

$$= \underline{\hspace{3cm}}$$

Interpretation. Results should be interpreted according to Table 4-5.

3-minute shuttle run

This test and the one that follows may give some indication of cardiovascular endurance even though they are performed for short periods of time.

Description of test. The 3-minute shuttle run is a simple test involving speed, agility, and cardiovascular endurance. Each student runs continuously for 3 minutes back and forth across a badminton court. Each time across the court, the subject touches the outside doubles line with one foot (Fig. 4-2). The aim is to cross the court as many times as possible during the 3-minute period. Each time the subject returns to the starting position, he has scored an additional two laps—one across and one back. The number of single laps completed during the 3-minute time period is counted and recorded.

Results. The results should be recorded in the spaces provided for them.

Number of single laps _____

Distance across court   = 20 feet

Total distance covered =

Number of single laps × 20 feet

= _____ × 20 feet

= _____ feet

Interpretation. Results for the 3-minute shuttle run should be interpreted according to Table 4-6.

Fig. 4-2. Diagram showing the layout of a badminton court. The two outside lines are identified as *A* and *B*. The subject runs across the court and touches one of these lines with his foot. He then turns and runs to the opposite side and touches the other line with his foot. This would constitute the completion of two single laps.

Table 4-6. Classification of scores obtained for the 3-minute shuttle run

Classification	Men (number of single laps)	Women (number of single laps)
Very poor	Less than 65	Less than 53
Poor	65-69	54-58
Average	70-82	59-70
Good	83-87	71-76
Excellent	More than 88	More than 77

Table 4-7. Classification of scores obtained for the 1-minute lateral jump test

Classification	Men (number of single jumps)	Women (number of single jumps)
Very poor	Less than 134	Less than 130
Poor	135-155	131-146
Average	156-180	147-173
Good	181-198	174-183
Excellent	More than 199	More than 184

1-minute lateral jump test

Description of test. The 1-minute lateral jump test is another simple test involving speed, agility, and cardiovascular endurance. Keeping both feet together, each subject jumps laterally across a line on the floor as many times as possible during a 1-minute period of time. Each time both feet cross the line, this counts as one jump, so that each time the subject returns to the starting position he has an additional two jumps. The aim is to score as many jumps as possible. This can be achieved by jumping close to the line, by bending the knees slightly, and by using the arms to maintain balance.

Results. The results should be recorded in the spaces provided for them.

Number of single jumps completed in 1 minute _____

Interpretation. The results of the 1-minute lateral jump test should be interpreted according to Table 4-7.

REFERENCES

1. Balke, B.: A simple field test for the assessment of physical fitness, Washington, D. C., 1963, U. S. Government Printing Office, p. 1.
2. Cooper, K. H.: Aerobics, New York, 1968, M. Evans and Company, Inc.
3. Doolittle, T. L., et al.: Reliability of the 12-minute run-walk test when employed with adolescent girls, Paper read at the American Association of Health, Physical Education, and Recreation, National Convention, Boston, Mass., April, 1969.
4. Doolittle, T. L., and Bigbee, R.: Twelve-minute run-walk: a test of cardiorespiratory fitness of adolescent boys, Research Quarterly **39:**491, Oct., 1968.
5. Karvonen, M. J.: Effects of vigorous exercise on the heart. In Rosenbaum, F. F., and Belknap, E. L., editors: Work and the heart, New York, 1959, Paul B. Hoeber, Inc.

Name _____ Date _____

Day and hour laboratory section meets _____

Laboratory instructor _____

CARDIOVASCULAR EVALUATION
Summary of results

Heart rate reliability

1. _____ beats/min

2. _____ beats/min

3. _____ beats/min

4. _____ beats/min

Step test data

1. Time of stepping _____ seconds

2. Recovery heart rate (1-1½ min of recovery)

   _____ beats/½ min

3. Physical efficiency index _____

4. Cardiovascular classification _____

12-minute field test

1. Number of laps completed _____

2. Distance of one lap _____ feet

3. Total distance covered _____ miles

4. Cardiovascular classification _____

3-minute shuttle run

1. Number of single laps completed _____

2. Distance across court _____

3. Total distance covered _____

4. Cardiovascular classification _____

1-minute lateral jump test

1. Number of single jumps _____

2. Cardiovascular classification _____

1½-mile run

1. Time to complete 1½ miles _____ min

   _____ sec

2. Cardiovascular classification _____

Name _____ Date _____

Day and hour laboratory section meets _____

Laboratory instructor _____

CARDIOVASCULAR PROFILE CHART FOR MEN

Percentile rank indicates the percentage of students whose score was less than your score. For example, if your physical efficiency index on the Harvard step test was 95, you would have a percentile rank of 70, based on the scores for the 16-inch bench. This would mean that you performed better than 70% of the students who took this test.

Directions

Circle the score closest to that obtained by you on each test. Connect each circle by a line so that comparisons may be made among the four tests.

Percentile rank	Harvard step test (physical efficiency index)		12-minute run (miles)	3-minute shuttle run (number of single laps)	1-minute lateral jump test (number of single jumps)	1½ mile run (min:sec)
	16-inch bench	20-inch bench				
95	115	100	1.92	89	206	9:20
90	108	94	1.84	86	198	9:42
80	101	87	1.74	83	188	10:18
70	95	82	1.67	80	181	10:42
60	90	78	1.62	78	176	11:06
50	86	74	1.56	76	170	11:30
40	82	70	1.50	74	164	12:00
30	77	66	1.45	72	159	12:24
20	71	61	1.38	69	152	13:12
10	64	54	1.26	66	142	14:18
5	57	48	1.20	63	134	15:00
Mean	86.0	74.0	1.56	76.0	170.0	11:30
SD	17.5	11.1	.22	8.0	22.0	1:12

Name _____ Date _____

Day and hour laboratory section meets _____

Laboratory instructor _____

CARDIOVASCULAR PROFILE CHART FOR WOMEN

Percentile rank indicates the percentage of students whose score was less than your score. For example, if your physical efficiency index on the Harvard step test is 66, you have a percentile rank of 30. This means that you performed better than only 30% of the students who took the test.

Directions

Circle the score closest to that obtained by you on each test. Connect each circle by a line so that comparisons may be made among the four tests.

Percentile rank	Harvard step test (physical efficiency index)	12-minute run (miles)	3-minute shuttle run (number of single laps)	1-minute lateral jump test (number of single jumps)	1½ mile run (min:sec)
95	100	1.45	78	186	12:24
90	94	1.39	75	180	12:57
80	87	1.33	72	172	13:30
70	82	1.27	69	167	14:10
60	78	1.23	67	162	14:36
50	74	1.20	65	158	15:00
40	70	1.17	63	154	15:24
30	66	1.13	61	149	15:50
20	61	1.07	58	144	16:48
10	54	1.01	55	136	17:48
5	48	.95	52	130	19:00
Mean	74.0	1.20	65.0	158.0	15:00
SD	11.1	.15	8.0	17.0	1:30

CHAPTER **5**

Strength

What do you know about strength?

T F

☐ ☐ **1.** Overall strength may best be determined by administration of the grip strength test.

☐ ☐ **2.** Strength of the abdominal muscles can best be measured by the number of bent-leg sit-ups a person can perform in 1 minute.

☐ ☐ **3.** Any person who lifts weights regularly will become muscle bound because high resistance exercises limit range of motion.

☐ ☐ **4.** Strength may best be measured as the maximal amount of force that a muscle group can exert once only.

☐ ☐ **5.** Isotonic exercises are far superior to isometric exercises for the development of strength.

☐ ☐ **6.** Strength is really a synonym for muscular endurance.

☐ ☐ **7.** An isotonic contraction involves exerting muscular force against an immovable object.

☐ ☐ **8.** Holding a 20-pound weight at arm's length for 10 seconds exemplifies an isometric contraction.

☐ ☐ **9.** To improve strength one should use light weights and complete as many repetitions as possible.

Strength may be defined as the maximal one-effort force that can be exerted against a resistance. For many years this was regarded as the symbol of physical fitness, and many of the physical fitness tests were simply strength tests. A person with well-developed musculature and a good physique was considered to exhibit good physical fitness. However, it should be kept in mind that fitness should not be based on physical appearance but on the functional capacity of the individual to perform work and to supply the necessary energy. The importance attached to the development of strength in increasing one's physical fitness level has declined in recent years. However, it cannot be denied that a minimal level of strength is necessary, for without this it would be impossible to carry out the tasks that are necessary each day. All movement is to a degree dependent on a certain minimal level of strength. A person with poorly developed musculature will find it difficult to maintain an upright posture.

It should also be emphasized that a person who is engaged in hard physical work is going to need a much higher degree of strength than a person who has an office job and spends much of his time sitting behind a desk.

MEASUREMENT OF STRENGTH

Strength is measured correctly by determining the maximal force that a muscle or muscle group can exert once and once only. It is not properly measured by how many times an exercise can be performed or how long an individual can perform a given exercise. These are both measures of muscular endurance and are not measures of strength. For example, it is commonly thought that the number of push-ups or pull-ups is an adequate measure of strength. These tests actually measure muscular endurance. Grip strength is probably the most commonly used measurement (Fig. 5-1). The subject squeezes the hand dynamometer and exerts a maximal force once and once only as the musculature contracts forcedly. The force exerted is recorded on the dial.

Fig. 5-1. Measurement of grip strength.

To evaluate strength, many tests must be administered. This is because strength is not a general component but is specific to a particular muscle or group of muscles. Just because one muscle group is well developed does not mean that other groups will be similarly developed. This is known as the principle of specificity. A gymnast, for example, who works on the parallel bars is more likely to have well-developed musculature of the upper body, whereas his muscular development in the legs may be classified as only normal.

DEVELOPMENT OF STRENGTH

Strength may be developed by either isometric or isotonic exercises, or a combination of both.

Isometric training

An *isometric contraction* may be defined as a contraction that occurs when a force is exerted against an immovable object. The length of the muscle does not shorten as a static contraction occurs. An example of this type of contraction would be the measurement of back strength (Fig. 5-2). In this test and other tests like this the subject executes a maximal exertion against an immovable bar, and the force is registered on a gauge.

Isometric training was first made popular in the early 1950s through the research of Hettinger and Mueller,[2] two German physiologists. They showed strength gains from 33% to 181% with isometric exercises performed once daily for 6 seconds per day 5 days a week.

The advantages of isometric training are obvious. A minimal amount of equipment and time is necessary, and large groups of students can participate at the same time. Also these exercises are usually easy to follow, and undue fatigue is avoided.

The major limitation is that isometric exercises can develop strength at only one specific point in the range of motion, whereas with isotonic exercises a *full* range of motion is possi-

Fig. 5-2. Measurement of back strength—an example of an isometric contraction.

ble. Also, if a subject cannot see any work being performed, maintaining motivation is often difficult.

The most recent research of Mueller and Rohmert[3] indicates that maximal gains in strength can be achieved by holding a maximal contraction for 5 seconds, five to ten times a

Fig. 5-3. Demonstration of position for the hand push (left) and the elbow push (right). Both of these are examples of isometric exercises.

day. They also suggest that these contractions be applied at varying points in the range of motion rather than all at the same angle.

Examples of several isometric exercises that require no equipment follow. These are but a few of the isometric exercises that can be designed to develop the strength and muscular endurance of different muscle groups.

Elbow push. The subject stands with back touching the wall, elbows at shoulder height and also touching the wall, and forearms flexed and hands beneath the chin with palms down. The elbows are pressed against the wall, as a maximum contraction is held for 5 seconds (Fig. 5-3).

Hand push. The subject stands with the palms together and the elbows raised to shoulder height. The palms are pressed together as hard as possible, and the maximal contraction is then held (Fig. 5-3).

V-sit. For the V-sit exercise the subject sits on the floor, places the hands on the hips, and leans backward until the trunk forms an angle of approximately 45° with the floor. Keeping the legs straight, the feet are raised approximately 12 to 20 inches from the floor as a V position is assumed and then held for a given period of time (Fig. 11-3).

Muscle-maker. The subject flexes the forearm until the elbow joint forms approximately a right angle. The biceps muscle in the front of the upper arm is then contracted maximally, and this contraction is held.

Sit-up. The subject assumes a supine (face-up) position on the floor with the legs out straight in front of him. The upper part of the body is raised off the floor as he sits up, so that the trunk is at a right angle to the legs. A partner straddles the legs and pushes against the chest or elbows (Fig. 5-4). Maximal force is exerted against the force of the partner.

Isotonic training

An *isotonic contraction* occurs when the muscle contracts and shortens and movement takes place. Any time a person lifts a weight through a range of motion (Fig. 5-5), an isotonic contraction takes place. Most common ex-

Fig. 5-4. Demonstration of the position to be held for the isometric sit-up.

Fig. 5-5. Performance of a two-arm curl—an example of an isotonic contraction as the weight is lifted through a range of movement.

Fig. 5-6. Mean strength results from six groups, each involved with a different training method. (Data from Berger.[1])

Table 5-1. Results of grip strength tests (pounds)

	Trial 1	Trial 2	Best
Dominant hand			
Nondominant hand			

ercises, such as calisthenics and weight lifting, involve isotonic contractions as shortening and lengthening take place. To bring about maximal gains in strength with isotonic methods, few repetitions need to be performed, and the resistance needs to be high. It has been shown that maximal gains in strength occur when the number of repetitions ranges from four to eight and the maximal weight that can be lifted for this number of times is used (Fig. 5-6).

The major advantage of isotonic exercises is that the work can be performed through the full range of motion. Also the individual can see the work being done, which appears to increase the motivation of the participant.

LABORATORY EXPERIENCE
Grip strength

A hand dynamometer is used to measure the force of the hand's muscular contraction. It is placed in the palm of the hand with the dial facing the palm. It is then squeezed as tightly as possible, with the hand and the arm away from the body. It is not permitted for the hand or the upper arm to push against any other object or against any part of the body. The score is recorded to the nearest pound in Table 5-1.

To find out how your best score compares with scores from other college students you should circle the score closest to yours on the profile chart at the end of this section.

Weight lifting exercises for strength or muscular endurance

Two-arm curl. This exercise is designed for the development of the flexors of the forearm. The subject stands with the feet shoulder width apart in an upright position. A barbell is held with the palms-forward grip and the arms extended. With the elbows close to the body, the bar is curled to the shoulder-neck area and re-

Fig. 5-7. Starting **(A)** and finishing **(B)** positions for two-arm curl exercise.

Fig. 5-8. Starting **(A)** and finishing **(B)** positions for bench press exercise.

Fig. 5-9. Starting **(A)** and finishing **(B)** positions for lateral machine pull-down exercise.

turned to the starting position. This constitutes one complete repetition (Fig. 5-7).

Bench press. This exercise is for the development of the chest and shoulders and the extensors of the forearm. The subject lies flat on a bench with the knees bent and the feet flat on the floor. The barbell is held with the palms-forward grip at approximately the width of the shoulders. The bar is then pressed directly upward until the arms are fully extended; then it is returned to the starting position to complete one repetition (Fig. 5-8). The back may not be arched during this exercise but must remain in contact with the bench.

Lateral machine pull-down. This exercise is for the flexors of the forearm, the back, and the upper chest. The subject assumes a kneeling position and the bar is grasped with the palms-

forward grip as in Fig. 5-9. The bar is pulled down until it touches the base of the neck and then returned to the starting position to complete one repetition. The body must be kept straight throughout, and no jerking is allowed (Fig. 5-9.)

Upright rowing. This exercise is designed for the development of the flexors of the forearm and the shoulders and back. The subject assumes a standing position and grasps the bar with the palms-down grip and the hands approximately 4 inches apart (Fig. 5-10). The bar is then raised until it touches the chin and is then lowered back to the starting position to complete one repetition. The bar must be kept close to the body, and the elbows must remain higher than the hands throughout the lift (Fig. 5-10).

Fig. 5-10. Starting **(A)** and finishing **(B)** positions for upright rowing exercise.

Fig. 5-11. Starting **(A)** and finishing **(B)** positions for quadriceps lift exercise.

Fig. 5-12. Starting **(A)** and finishing **(B)** positions for the leg curl exercise.

Quadriceps lift. This exercise is designed for the development of the front of the thigh and the extensors of the lower part of the leg. The subject assumes a sitting position with the lower legs at right angles to the thighs and the front of the ankles against the bar (Fig. 5-11).The legs are extended until they are parallel with the floor and then returned to the starting position. The upper body must remain in an upright position throughout (Fig. 5-11).

Leg curl. This exercise is designed for the flexors of the lower part of the leg, mainly the hamstring muscle group. The subject lies face downward with the legs extended and the backs of the heels against the bar (Fig. 5-12). The feet are then lifted upward until they touch the buttocks or are positioned immediately above the buttocks. They are then returned to the starting position (Fig. 5-12).

Curl up. This exercise is for the development

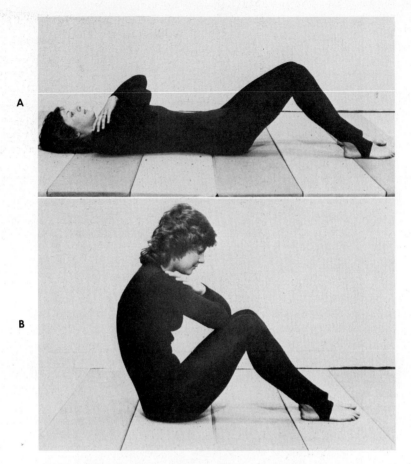

Fig. 5-13. Starting **(A)** and finishing **(B)** positions for the curl-up exercise.

of the abdominal muscles. The subject lies flat on the floor with the knees bent, forming an angle of approximately 90° and the feet flat on the floor. The hands are folded over the chest. The subject curls up until the elbows touch the thighs and then returns to the starting position. It is important to avoid jerky movements and to start by bending the head forward slowly (Fig. 5-13).

Determination of strength for these tests

To determine the strength for each of these areas, a trial-and-error method must be used to determine the maximal amount of weight that can be lifted once and once only for each of these exercises. This is referred to as one-repetition maximum (1 RM).

REFERENCES

1. Berger, R. A., Optimum repetitions for the development of strength. Research Quarterly **33**:334-338, 1962.
2. Hettinger, T., and Mueller, E. A.: Die Muskelleistung und Muskeltrainerung. Arbeitsphysiologie **15**:111, 1953.
3. Mueller, E. A., and Rohmert, W.: Die Geschwindigkeit der Muselkraftzunahme bei isometrischen Trainierung, Int. Z. Angew. Physiol. **19**:403, 1963.

Name _____ Date _____

Day and hour laboratory section meets _____

Laboratory instructor _____

GRIP STRENGTH PROFILE CHART

Percentile rank	Men		Women	
	Dominant hand (pounds)	Nondominant hand (pounds)	Dominant hand (pounds)	Nondominant hand (pounds)
95	159	147	88	83
90	152	140	84	79
80	144	132	79	74
70	138	126	76	71
60	133	121	73	68
50	128	116	70	65
40	123	111	67	62
30	118	106	64	59
20	112	100	61	56
10	104	92	56	51
5	97	85	52	47
Mean	128.0	116.0	70.0	65.0
SD	19.0	19.0	11.0	11.0

Name _____ Date _____

Day and hour laboratory section meets _____

Laboratory instructor _____

SUMMARY SHEET FOR STRENGTH TESTS

Grip strength

Dominant hand: Trial 1 _____ pounds
                             } Best score _____ pounds
                    Trial 2 _____ pounds

Nondominant hand: Trial 1 _____ pounds
                             } Best score _____ pounds
                    Trial 2 _____ pounds

For the following tests, the maximum weight that could be lifted once is recorded.

Two-arm curl	_____ pounds	**Quad lift**	_____ pounds
Bench press	_____ pounds	**Leg curl**	_____ pounds
Lateral machine pull-down	_____ pounds	**Curl up**	_____ pounds
Upright rowing	_____ pounds		

CHAPTER 6

Muscular endurance

What do you know about muscular endurance?

T F

☐ ☐ **1.** Muscular endurance may be measured by the length of time a particular muscle group can sustain a contraction.

☐ ☐ **2.** Muscular endurance is the maximal amount of force a muscle or muscle group can exert once only.

☐ ☐ **3.** Sit-ups should be performed with straight legs for the development of abdominal muscular endurance.

☐ ☐ **4.** The limiting factors for a muscular endurance task are associated with the heart and circulatory system.

T F

☐ ☐ **5.** A muscular endurance task performed to exhaustion will result in a near maximal heart rate.

☐ ☐ **6.** To improve muscular endurance by weight training, keep the number of repetitions constant and increase the resistance each week.

☐ ☐ **7.** Muscular endurance can be developed by isometric methods in addition to isotonic methods.

Table 6-1. Muscular endurance tests

Test	Suggested for men	Suggested for women
Bent-leg sit-up	Yes	Yes
Push-up	Yes	No
Static push-up	Yes	Yes
Pull-up	Yes	No
Flexed-arm hang	No	Yes
Burpee	Yes	Yes
Bench jump	Yes	Yes

Muscular endurance may be defined as the ability of the muscles to apply force repeatedly or to sustain a contraction for a period of time. Another definition is ''the ability to perform work continually involving local muscular effort.'' For example, if one wishes to measure the endurance of the abdominal muscles, this could be done by determining how many times they can contract within a given time period (bent-leg sit-ups) or how long they can sustain a given contraction (V-sit position).

The longer a muscle can contract without fatigue or the greater the number of repetitions that can be performed before fatigue, the higher the muscular endurance. With this type of work the limiting factor is localized in the muscle group itself, and the circulatory system is usually not taxed to its fullest capacity. Consider, for example, the performance of the simple pull-up. If a student is instructed to do as many pull-ups as possible, a point is reached finally where he is unable to perform any more. He has reached his limit as far as the functional capacity of the muscle group involved is concerned. If the heart rate were monitored throughout, it would show that it is still far from maximal, indicating that the heart and circulatory system are not the limiting factors as far as the task is concerned.

MEASUREMENT OF MUSCULAR ENDURANCE

Muscular endurance is also specific to each of the muscle groups, and because of this many tests are necessary if a complete evaluation of this physical fitness component is to be made. Several of these tests are identified in Table 6-1, followed by a description of the administrative procedures.

Bent-leg sit-up

The bent-leg sit-up is a measure of the muscular endurance of the abdominal muscles. These muscles are very important in maintaining good posture. The subject lies on the back with the fingers interlocked behind the neck. Both feet are placed flat on the floor, and the knees are flexed, forming an angle of approximately 90°. With feet held firmly in place, the subject sits up so that at least one elbow touches one knee (Fig. 6-1). Each elbow *may* touch each knee if the subject desires; however, the most efficient way is to touch one elbow to one knee and to alternate this each time. Each time the subject returns to the starting position, the fingers at the back of the head must come in contact with the floor before the next sit-up is attempted. This process is repeated as many times as possible during a 1-minute period.

Results. Number of sit-ups in 1 minute _____.

Sitting tuck

To develop the muscular endurance of the abdominal muscles, the sitting tuck exercises may be preferred to bent-leg sit-ups (Fig. 6-2). The subject assumes a supine position with arms extended over the head. The subject then

Fig. 6-1. Bent-leg sit-up in test of muscular endurance.

Fig. 6-2. Finishing position for sitting tuck exercise.

curls up in a sitting position while bringing the arms and hands up to grasp the knees, which are also flexed simultaneously.

Results. Number of sitting tucks _____ .

Push-up (men only)

The push-up is a measure of the endurance of the muscle group concerned with extension of the forearm. The largest muscle of this group is the triceps. The subject assumes a prone position on the floor with hands directly under the shoulder joints, legs straight and together, and toes tucked under so that they are in contact with the floor. The subject then pushes with the arms until they are fully extended. The body is then lowered until the chin or chest touches the floor. At this point there should be a straight line from the head to the toes. All of this movement must be performed by the arms and shoulders and not by any other part of the body. This movement is repeated as many times as possible. There is no time limit to this test, but the push-ups must be performed continuously.

Results. Number of push-ups _____.

Static push-up

This is a measure of the endurance of the muscle group concerned with the extension of the forearm and is an alternate test to the push-up for men. It is intended for women and is preferred to the modified push-up because of the ease of administration and because it is much easier to standardize procedures.

From a straight-arm, front leaning position, with the hands directly under the shoulders, the subject lowers the body until the elbows are flexed to 90° or less. The subject holds this position as long as possible. The test is terminated and the time recorded when any part of the body other than the hands or toes touches the floor or when the body is not maintained in a parallel position to the floor.

Results. Time for static push-up _____ min _____ sec.

Pull-up (men only)

The pull-up is primarily a measure of the endurance of the muscle group responsible for flexion of the forearm. The major muscle of this group is the biceps brachii or, as it is commonly referred to, the biceps. The subject grasps the horizontal bar with both hands, palms facing forward. The "dead hang" position is assumed, with arms fully extended and feet off the ground. The body is raised until the chin is above the top of the bar and is then lowered until the arms are fully extended. The process is repeated until the subject can no longer raise his chin above the bar. The knees may not be raised nor is kicking permitted in an attempt to perform more chinnings.

Results. Number of pull-ups _____.

Flexed-arm hang (women only)

This test measures the endurance of the flexors of the forearm. Each subject must use the overhand grip with the palms facing forward. The subject then raises the body off the floor to a position where the chin is level with the bar. This position is maintained for as long as possible. Time is stopped when the chin cannot be maintained level with the bar.

Results. Time for flexed-arm hang _____ min _____ sec.

Modified pull-up (women only)

In the modified pull-up the bar is adjusted to the height of the sternum, and the feet remain in contact with the floor throughout. The subject grips the bar with the palms forward and slides her feet under the bar until the arms form a right angle with the body. The weight must rest on the heels as the subject attempts to pull up, so that the chin or forehead touches the bar with the body held straight. This is attempted as many times as possible.

Results. Number of modified pull-ups _____.

Burpee

The burpee is a test of muscular endurance involving many large muscle groups. Rapid movements that involve changes in the body position are stressed. The subject stands at attention with feet together and hands at the sides. The squat position is then assumed with the hands placed on the floor adjacent to the feet. The legs are thrust to the rear as the subject assumes the front support position, and at this point the body must be perfectly straight. The feet are brought back to the hands as the squat position is again assumed, and the final step is back to the standing position. As many repetitions as possible are performed in a 1-minute time period.

Results. Number of burpees in 1 minute _____.

Table 6-2. Muscular endurance tests using weights

Exercise	Body weight	Percent of body weight	Resistance to be used	Repetitions completed	Points earned
Two-arm curl	_____	$33^1/_3$	_____	_____	_____
Bench press	_____	$66^2/_3$	_____	_____	_____
Lateral machine pull-down	_____	$66^2/_3$	_____	_____	_____
Upright rowing	_____	$33^1/_3$	_____	_____	_____
Quadriceps lift	_____	$66^2/_3$	_____	_____	_____
Leg curl	_____	$33^1/_3$	_____	_____	_____
Curl up	_____	14	_____	_____	_____

Bench jump

The bench jump is designed to determine the muscular endurance of the muscles of the lower extremity. A 16-inch bench is used, and each subject attempts to jump up to the bench as many times as possible during a 1-minute period. If he is unable to jump he may step up; however, this takes more time. His arms may swing freely, but he is not permitted to push off his thighs when stepping up. One repetition is counted each time both his feet are planted on the bench and he returns to the floor.

Results. Number of bench jumps in 1 minute

_____.

ALTERNATE MUSCULAR ENDURANCE EVALUATION USING WEIGHTS OR WEIGHT MACHINE

The following method of evaluation of muscular endurance is adapted from Allsen, Harrison, and Vance[1] and is based on the earlier work of DiGennaro.[2] The seven exercises used and the amount of weight used for each person for each exercise are summarized in Table 6-2. It should be noted that these exercises are the same exercises described in detail in the preceding chapter on strength (Chapter 5). The maximum number of repetitions for men is 17 and

Table 6-3. Evaluation of muscular endurance tests

Repetitions		Points	Muscular endurance category
Men	Women		
0-3	0-2	5	Very poor
4	3	7	Poor
5-8	4-7	9	Fair
9-11	8-10	11	Good
12-16	11-14	13	Very good
17	15	15	Excellent

Table 6-4. Overall muscular endurance classification (total points for all seven tests)

Points	Category
35-48	Very poor
49-62	Poor
63-76	Fair
77-90	Good
91-104	Very good
105	Excellent

for women is 15. The resistance in each case is a designated percentage of the body weight of each subject.

Allsen, Harrison, and Vance[1] recommend the following point scale for evaluating each exercise (Table 6-3).

They further suggest that to get an indication of a person's overall muscular endurance the points gained for all seven exercises are added and they should be interpreted according to Table 6-4.

REFERENCES

1. Allsen, P., Harrison, J. M., and Vance, B.: Fitness for life: an individualized approach, Dubuque, Iowa, 1975, Wm. C. Brown Company, Publishers.
2. DiGennaro, J.: Individualized exercise and optimal physical fitness, Philadelphia, 1974, Lea & Febiger.

Name _____ Date _____

Day and hour laboratory section meets _____

Laboratory instructor _____

MUSCULAR ENDURANCE PROFILE CHART
Directions

Circle the score closest to the one obtained by you on each test. Connect each circle by a line so that comparisons may be made among the nine tests.

Men

Percentile rank	Bent-leg sit-ups (1 min max)	Push-ups	Static push-ups	Pull-ups	Burpees (1 min max)	Bench jumps
95	50	53	114	14	40	38
90	47	49	111	12	38	36
80	44	44	106	10	36	34
70	41	41	102	9	35	33
60	39	38	100	8	33	31
50	37	35	97	7	32	30
40	35	32	94	6	31	29
30	33	29	92	5	29	27
20	30	26	88	4	28	26
10	27	21	83	2	26	24
5	24	17	80	0	24	22
Mean	37.0	35.0	97.0	7.0	32.0	29.8
SD	8.0	8.0	11.8	4.0	4.7	4.7

Women

Percentile rank	Bent-leg sit-ups (1 min max)	Static push-ups	Flexed-arm hang	Modified pull-ups	Burpees (1 min max)	Bench jumps
95	36	38	34	43	30	28
90	33	35	28	40	28	26
80	30	32	19	36	26	24
70	28	30	14	33	24	22
60	26	28	10	30	23	21
50	24	26	8	28	22	20
40	22	24	6	26	21	19
30	20	22	4	23	20	18
20	18	20	2	20	18	16
10	15	17	1	16	16	14
5	12	14	0	13	14	12
Mean	24.0	26.2	8.1	28.0	22.0	20.1
SD	7.4	7.6	2.5	9.4	4.7	4.7

Name _____ **Date** _____

Day and hour laboratory section meets _____

Laboratory instructor _____

SUMMARY SHEET FOR MUSCULAR ENDURANCE TESTS

Men	Number	Percentile
Bent-leg sit-ups	_____	_____
Push-ups	_____	_____
Pull-ups	_____	_____
Burpees	_____	_____
Static push-ups	_____	_____
Bench jumps	_____	_____

Women	Number	Percentile
Bent-leg sit-ups	_____	_____
Flexed-arm han	_____	_____
Static push-ups	_____	_____
Modified pull-up	_____	_____
Burpees	_____	_____
Bench jumps	_____	_____

CHAPTER 7

Flexibility

What do you know about flexibility?

T F

☐ ☐ **1.** Flexibility can be defined as the maximal range of movement possible at each joint.

☐ ☐ **2.** The sit and reach test will give an adequate indication of overall flexibility.

☐ ☐ **3.** Inactive persons are usually less flexible than active people.

☐ ☐ **4.** College-age women are much more flexible than college-age men.

☐ ☐ **5.** Flexibility is specific to each joint.

☐ ☐ **6.** Possession of adequate flexibility may result in a reduction in the incidence of low back pain.

Flexibility may be defined as the functional capacity of the joints to move through a full range of movement. The length of the muscles, ligaments, and tendons largely determines the amount of movement possible at each joint.

It appears as though inactive persons are usually less flexible than persons who are more active. This may be caused by the fact that inactive individuals spend much more time sitting, in which case certain muscle groups are constantly in the flexed position. For example, when a sitting position is assumed, there is usually flexion at the knee joint, at the hip joint, and at the elbow joint. The maintenance of this position for extended periods of time results in these muscles becoming much shorter than they should be. Additional stretching exercises are often necessary if adequate flexibility is to result and if these muscles are to retain their nor-mal length. Without an adequate amount of flexibility one cannot possibly function at his optimal level.

DEVELOPMENT OF FLEXIBILITY

Maintaining adequate flexibility seems to depend on the amount and intensity of movement of the body parts through complete ranges of motion several times a day. For those whose daily living habits do not result in such movement, it is advisable to participate daily in selected exercises that stress movement of the joints through a full range of motion. Exercises that are performed slowly appear to be more beneficial and less likely to result in injury than exercises that involve bobbing, bouncing, or jerky movements. Isometric exercises can also be used effectively for the development of flexibility.

Fig. 7-1. Sit-and-reach test of flexibility.

MEASUREMENT OF FLEXIBILITY

Again it should be stressed that flexibility is not a general component of physical fitness but is specific to each joint. It is therefore not possible to measure flexibility by just one test. Each movement that is possible at each joint must be measured if all aspects of flexibility are to be evaluated.

Leighton[1] has developed an instrument, called a Flexometer, for the measurement of movement at each joint. Use of this instrument is one of the best methods for the determination of joint flexibility. A number of specific tests have been developed for classroom use when a

Flexometer is not available. Three of the more commonly used tests are described on the following pages.

Trunk flexion—sit and reach

The degree of trunk flexion will depend on the length of the trunk extensor muscles of the back and also the hamstring muscles. The subject assumes a sitting position with the knees fully extended and the bottom of the feet against the lower board of the bleachers. The hands and arms are stretched forward as far as possible, and this position is held for 3 seconds (Fig. 7-1). A ruler is used to measure the distance in

Fig. 7-2. Stand-and-reach test of flexibility.

front of or beyond the edge of the bench. Measures in front are negative, whereas measures beyond are positive. This test may also be taken by standing on a bench and reaching down as far as possible (Fig. 7-2).

Results. Trunk flexion—sit and reach _____ inches (be sure to indicate either + or −).

Trunk extension

The trunk extension test is a measure of the range of motion when the back is arched from the prone position. The subject lies facedown on the floor with a partner holding the buttocks and legs down. The fingers are interlocked and the head and shoulders are raised as far as pos-

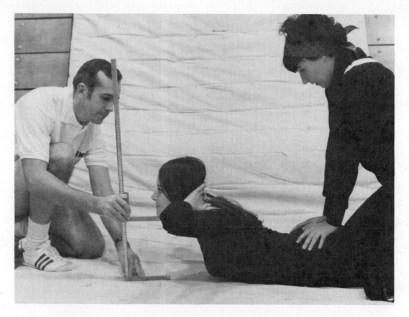

Fig. 7-3. Trunk-extension test of flexibility.

Fig. 7-4. Shoulder-lift test of flexibility.

sible from the floor (Fig. 7-3). The distance is measured from floor to chin.

Results. Trunk extension _____ inches.

Shoulder lift

The shoulder lift test measures the range of flexion at the shoulder joint. The subject lies facedown on the floor with his arms parallel and holding a ruler in his hands. The chin and forehead must remain on the floor while the ruler is raised as high as possible with the arms straight. The wrists may not be bent upward in an attempt to achieve a higher score (Fig. 7-4). This position is held for 3 seconds, and the distance from floor to lower edge of the ruler is measured.

Results. Shoulder lift _____ inches.

FLEXIBILITY EXERCISES

Before beginning any exercise program it is important to warm up adequately and to perform several stretching exercises. Each must be performed by moving through a full range of motion. Bouncy, jerky movements should be avoided. Following are some exercises that can be used adequately for stretching and warm-up. Each position should be held for 6 to 10 seconds and repeated five times.

Standing hamstring stretcher

One leg should be raised and the back of the foot placed on a solid object, such as a table or chair, with the toe pointing forward or up. The subject should reach and lean toward the raised foot as far as possible (Fig. 7-5).

Sitting hamstring stretcher

The subject should sit on the floor with legs straight and feet about 12 inches apart, bend forward slowly at the waist, grasp an ankle with both hands. The head should then be lowered to assume a position as close to the knee as possible (Fig. 7-6).

Fig. 7-5. Position for standing hamstring stretcher.

Fig. 7-6. Position for sitting hamstring stretcher.

Fig. 7-7. Position for low back stretcher.

Fig. 7-8. Position for hurdler's stretch exercise.

Low back stretcher

The subject should lie faceup with the knees straight. One leg is pulled up to the chest as far as possible while grasping the lower leg. At the same time the head and shoulders are raised toward the knees (Fig. 7-7).

Hurdler's stretch

After assuming the position illustrated, the subject should reach forward with both hands and grasp the ankle or foot that is extended in front (Fig. 7-8).

Other stretching exercises described in Chapter 12 include the following:
1. Hip raiser exercise (Fig. 12-1).
2. Lateral leg raise (Fig. 12-2).
3. Sprinter exercise (Fig. 12-6).

REFERENCE

1. Leighton, J. R.: Instrument and technic for measurement of range of joint motion. Archives of Physical Medicine and Rehabilitation **36:**571, Sept., 1955.

Name _____ **Date** _____

Day and hour laboratory section meets _____

Laboratory instructor _____

FLEXIBILITY PROFILE CHART

Percentile rank	Men			Women		
	Sit and reach (inches)	Trunk extension (inches)	Shoulder lift (inches)	Sit and reach (inches)	Trunk extension (inches)	Shoulder lift (inches)
95	+7.9	24	28	+6.8	22	27
90	+6.9	23	26	+5.9	20	25
80	+5.8	21	24	+4.9	18	22
70	+5.0	20	23	+4.1	17	21
60	+4.3	19	21	+3.6	16	19
50	+3.6	18	20	+3.0	15	18
40	+2.9	17	19	+2.4	14	17
30	+2.5	16	17	+1.9	13	15
20	+1.4	15	16	+0.9	12	14
10	+0.3	13	14	+0.1	10	11
5	−0.7	12	12	−0.8	8	9
Mean	+3.6	18.0	20.0	3.0	15.0	18.0
SD	+2.6	3.8	4.8	2.3	4.1	5.3

Name _____ **Date** _____

Day and hour laboratory section meets _____

Laboratory instructor _____

SUMMARY SHEET FOR FLEXIBILITY TESTS

1. Trunk flexion—sit and reach _____ inches

2. Trunk extension _____ inches

3. Shoulder lift _____ inches

CHAPTER 8

Exercise, diet, and weight control

What do you know about exercise, diet, and weight control?

T F

☐ ☐ **1.** An overweight person will also be obese.

☐ ☐ **2.** An obese person has a greatly reduced estimated life span.

☐ ☐ **3.** An overweight person is a person who is 10% or more above his desirable weight.

☐ ☐ **4.** The height/weight charts are the best method available for determination of ideal weight.

☐ ☐ **5.** Skinfold fat measurements are the best means of estimating body fat.

☐ ☐ **6.** Body weight is a dominant factor in determining the energy cost of an activity.

☐ ☐ **7.** Complete starvation for short periods of time is the quickest and best method of weight reduction.

☐ ☐ **8.** Exercise is a very poor weight reduction scheme because one needs to exercise too long to lose a pound of fat.

☐ ☐ **9.** A reduction in calorie intake together with an increase in daily activity is the best means by which a normal person can lose weight.

☐ ☐ **10.** Exercise is of little value in losing weight because if you exercise more you automatically eat more.

☐ ☐ **11.** Physical effort is essential to neutralize normal caloric intake.

☐ ☐ **12.** Obese individuals are less active than nonobese individuals.

One of the major health problems in the United States today is that of weight control. Recent data indicate that more than 60% of the adult population in this country is overweight, possibly for one or more of the following causes:

1. Higher standard of living
2. Increased mechanization
3. More leisure time
4. Less physical activity
5. Insufficient knowledge about weight control
6. Lack of motivation with regard to weight control

Allsen et al. have indicated that "if all the deaths from cancer were eliminated, two years would be added to man's life span, and if all the deaths related to obesity were removed, it is estimated that the life span would increase 7 years."[1]

To control weight effectively it is important to study carefully the mechanisms involved. This is most important when one considers the numbers of proposed easy methods available to control weight. Actually, many misconceptions concerning weight control are held by millions of persons.

The purpose of this chapter is to discuss certain common misconceptions pertaining to weight control and present factual information on the importance of exercise and diet.

DIFFERENTIATION BETWEEN AN OBESE AND AN OVERWEIGHT INDIVIDUAL

It is important to differentiate clearly between the terms *obese* and *overweight*. An *obese* person is one who has an excessive accumulation of body fat, which raises the question of what the normal or average amount of body fat is. In 1968 the average percentage of body fat to total weight for college freshmen was 12% to 13% for men and 20% to 21% for women. By 1975 these figures had increased to 15% to 16% for men and 25% to 26% for women.[19]

Mayer[12] suggests that if a quick estimate of obesity is desired, one can measure the amount of fat at the back of the upper arm in the area of the triceps muscle. He suggests that if this measurement exceeds 15 mm for men or 25 mm for women, the subject can be considered obese. It should be emphasized that these figures are normal or average figures for college-age men and women. They are not to be considered desirable, for many would agree that they are much higher than they should be.

An *overweight* person is one who is 10% or more above his desirable weight. Despite the recent national weight consciousness movement, it appears that the American adult population is steadily gaining weight, with an average increase of 14 pounds per capita over the past 10 years.[10]

Desirable weight has been defined as one at which each individual looks good, feels good, and can move efficiently. Originally, simple tables based on a person's height, age, and sex were used to determine the desirable weight. In 1963 the Metropolitan Life Insurance Company[15] introduced a new standard table based on different principles. The company recognized the undesirability of a continued increase in weight during adulthood past the termination of growth and realized, at least in theory, that persons vary according to body build. Weight ranges were then presented for three classes of frame size—small, medium, and large. However, determination of the category in which each individual was to be classified was apparently left to the subjective judgment of the examiner, since no criteria were presented for classification purposes.

A more recent classification has been prepared by the United States Department of Agriculture. Wrist girth is used to determine frame size, and subjects are classified according to Table 8-1. Tables 8-2 and 8-3 have been modified to indicate the *mean* desirable weight for each of the three classifications for designated heights.

Table 8-1. Frame classification according to wrist girth

Classification	Men (inches)	Women (inches)
Low (small)	5.6-6.7	4.6-5.5
Average (medium)	6.8-7.4	5.6-6.2
High (large)	7.5+	6.3-6.8

Table 8-2. Desirable weights for men 20 to 30 years old (weights listed without clothing according to height without shoes)*

Height (feet, inches)	Weight (pounds)		
	Low	Average	High
5-3	123	129	135
5-4	127	133	139
5-5	131	137	143
5-6	136	142	148
5-7	140	147	154
5-8	144	151	158
5-9	149	155	162
5-10	153	159	166
5-11	156	163	171
6-0	160	167	175
6-1	164	171	180
6-2	168	175	184
6-3	171	178	188

*From Food and your weight, Washington, D.C., 1973, U.S. Department of Agriculture, U.S. Government Printing Office.

Despite the fact that height-weight tables are used extensively, it should be realized that they do not measure the amount of excess weight that is in the form of fat or the amount that is in the form of muscle.

Most highly trained athletes, particularly football players, would be considered overweight by these standards. However, if these individuals are examined more closely, it can be shown that this excess weight is caused by muscular development and that the percentage of body fat is usually quite low. It is not how heavy a person is that is important but rather how much fat he carries.

Table 8-3. Desirable weights for women 20 to 30 years old (weights listed without clothing according to height without shoes)*

Height (feet, inches)	Weight (pounds)		
	Low	Average	High
5-0	104	109	114
5-1	108	112	117
5-2	111	115	120
5-3	114	118	123
5-4	117	122	127
5-5	120	125	130
5-6	124	129	134
5-7	128	132	137
5-8	131	136	141
5-9	135	140	146
5-10	138	144	150
5-11	142	148	155
6-0	146	152	159

*From Food and your weight, Washington, D.C., 1973, U.S. Department of Agriculture, U.S. Government Printing Office.

DETERMINATION OF PERCENT BODY FAT

It is difficult to measure accurately the fat content of the body. The best procedure is to use an underwater weighing technique to determine body density and to calculate percent body fat and lean body weight. However, this approach is not practical for mass testing and requires extensive equipment. Several alternate approaches have been adopted that attempt to estimate a person's percent body fat. These approaches use anthropometric measurements, body circumferences, or skinfold measurements along with previously established regression equations that predict the percentage of fat in the body. The most common method involves measuring the body fat thickness using skinfold calipers. An equation can then be used to estimate body density, lean body weight, or percent body fat.

Taking skinfold measurements requires practice to assure validity and reliability. The fol-

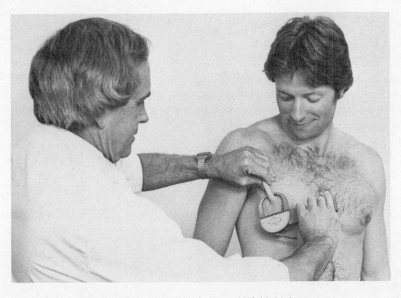

Fig. 8-1. Determination of chest skinfold thickness.

lowing suggestions for taking skinfold measurements should be followed:

1. Firmly grasp the fold of the skin between the left thumb and forefinger and lift up.
2. Place the contact surfaces of the calipers approximately 1.25 cm from the tips of the fingers.
3. Wait for approximately 2 seconds until the needle becomes relatively stable.
4. Read the measurement to the nearest 0.5 mm.
5. Three measurements should be taken at each site with at least two of these measurements equal. If not, additional measurements must be made until consistency is obtained.
6. All measurements should be made on the right side of the body.

The following are descriptions of the locations for skinfold measurements:

1. V_1–*Chest skinfold (men only):* Take a diagonal fold midway between the right nipple and the right axillary fold (Fig. 8-1).
2. V_2–*Subscapular skinfold:* Take a diagonal fold immediatly below the inferior

angle of the scapula. The natural fold will usually be away from the midline of the body and downwards (Fig. 8-2).

3. V_3–*Thigh skinfold:* With the subject seated on a table and the thigh in contact with the top of the table, take a vertical fold on the front of the thigh midway between the hip and knee joints (Fig. 8-3).
4. V_4–*Suprailiac skinfold:* Take a horizontal fold at the crest of the ilium (Fig. 8-4).
5. V_5–*Abdominal skinfold:* Take a horizontal fold on the right side adjacent to the umbilicus (Fig. 8-5).
6. V_6–*Triceps skinfold:* Take a fold running parallel to the length of the arm on the back of the arm midway between the shoulder and the elbow joint. The arm should be hanging naturally at the side in a relaxed position (Fig. 8-6).
7. V_7–*Midaxillary skinfold:* Take a vertical fold on the midaxillary line level with the lower part of the sternum (Fig. 8-7).

Two regression equations for predicting body density for men and women are summarized in Table 8-4. Any of the prediction equations can

Fig. 8-2. Determination of subscapular skinfold thickness.

Fig. 8-3. Determination of thigh skinfold thickness.

Fig. 8-4. Determination of iliac skinfold thickness.

Fig. 8-5. Determination of abdominal skinfold thickness.

Fig. 8-6. Determination of triceps skinfold thickness.

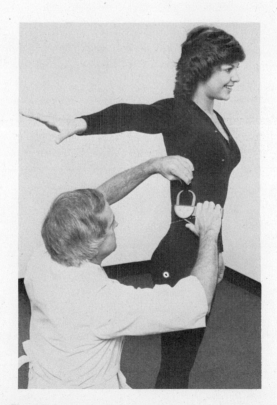

Fig. 8-7. Determination of midaxillary skinfold thickness.

Table 8-4. Regression equations for prediction of body density

Study	Sample	Regression equation
Men		
Pollock et al., 1976[16]	95 men ages 18-22	$BD = 1.09716 - 0.00065V_1 - 0.00055V_2 - 0.00080V_3$
Brozek and Keys, 1951[3]	133 men ages 18-26	$BD = 1.1017 - 0.000282V_2 - 0.000736V_1 - 0.000583V_6$
Women		
Pollock et al., 1975[17]	83 women ages 18-23	$BD = 1.0852 - 0.0008V_4 - 0.0011V_3$
Wilmore and Behnke, 1970[21]	128 women ages 18-48	$BD = 1.08543 - 0.000886V_5 - 0.00040V_3$

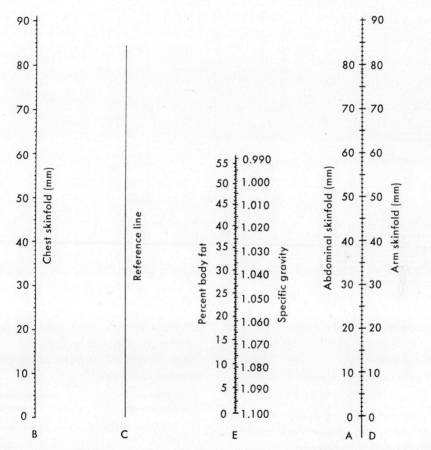

Fig. 8-8. Example of nomogram for conversion of skinfold thickness to specific gravity and percent fat in young men. Given: Abdominal skinfold 10 mm, chest skinfold 15 mm, and arm skinfold 20 mm. (1) With straight edge align abdominal value (10 mm) in column A with chest value (15 mm) in column B. (2) Place pin at point where straight edge crosses reference line C. (3) Pivot straight edge on pin to arm skinfold value (20 mm) in column D. (4) Read specific gravity (1.070) and percent body fat (14%) where straight edge crosses column E. Specific gravity = $1.1017 - 0.000282A - 0.000736B - 0.000883D$. (Brozek, J., and Keys, A.: British Journal of Nutrition **5**:194, 1951. Sample: 116 men, 18 to 26 years old.) Percent body fat = $100 (5.548/sp g - 5.044)$. (Rathbun, E. N., and Pace, N.: Journal of Biology and Chemistry **158**:667, 1945. Theoretically derived formula.) (Modified from Consolazio, C. F., et al.: Physiological measurements of metabolic functions in man, New York, 1963, McGraw-Hill Book Company. Used by permission of McGraw-Hill Book Company.)

Fig. 8-9. Nomogram for conversion of skinfold thickness to percent body fat for use with young women. (From Corbin, C., et al.: Concepts in physical education, Dubuque, Iowa, 1970. Used by permission of Wm. C. Brown Company, Publishers.)

be used to determine body density. The percentage of body fat can then be calculated using the following formula:

Percent body fat =
$$(4.95/\text{Body density} - 4.500) \times 100$$

The nomograms presented in Figs. 8-8 (men) and 8-9 (women) may also be used for determining the percentage of body fat.

ALTERNATE METHOD FOR ESTIMATING PERCENTAGE OF BODY FAT

An alternate method for estimating the percentage of body fat is to take two skinfold measurements, triceps and subscapular, and to calculate the sum of these two measurements. A percentile table for male and female college freshmen is presented in Table 8-5.

The obtained skinfold measurements can be recorded as follows:

Skinfold measurement	Obtained skinfold thickness (mm)
V_1 Chest (men only)	_____
V_2 Subscapular	_____
V_3 Thigh	_____
V_4 Suprailiac	_____
V_5 Abdominal	_____
V_6 Triceps	_____
V_7 Midaxillary	_____

This procedure has now been adopted by the American Association of Health, Physical Education, Recreation, and Dance for use in the

Table 8-5. Percentile table for interpretation of skinfold measurements for college freshmen[8]

Percentile rank	Sum of triceps and subscapular skinfold measurements	
	Male (mm)	Female (mm)
95	9	15
90	10	16
80	12	19
70	13	22
60	14	24
50	15	27
40	16	30
30	19	34
20	24	40
10	30	46
5	38	48

Table 8-6. Percentile table for college-age men for designated skinfold measurements*

Percentile	Chest	Triceps	Subscapular	Suprailiac	Abdominal	Thigh
95	2	4	2	2	6	4
90	5	5	5	5	8	6
80	8	6	8	8	10	8
70	11	7	11	11	14	10
60	14	8	14	14	18	12
50	17	9	17	17	22	14
40	20	11	20	21	27	17
30	23	13	23	25	32	20
20	26	15	26	29	37	23
10	29	17	29	33	42	26
5	32	19	32	37	47	29

*Adapted from Myers, C. R., editor: The Y's way to physical fitness, Columbus, Ohio, 1973, Rodale Press Inc., p. 48.

public schools with percentile tables available for ages 5 through 18. A percentile table for the various skinfold measurements for college-age men is presented in Table 8-6.

An arbitrary classification for percent body fat is presented in Table 8-7.

DETERMINATION OF PERCENT OVERWEIGHT
Determination of percent overweight using height-weight charts

1. Record your actual weight to the nearest pound.

   _____ pounds.

Table 8-7. Classification for determination of obesity

Classification	Men (percent)	Women (percent)
Very low	0-8	0-10
Low	9-12	11-15
Acceptable	13-15	16-20
Fat	16-17	21-25
Obese	18+	26+

2. Determine your frame size from your wrist girth.

   Wrist girth _____ inches.
   Frame size (see Table 8-1) _____.

3. Consult Table 8-2 (men) or 8-3 (women) to determine your desired weight.

   Desired weight _____.

4. Determine the difference between the desired weight and your actual weight.

   Difference _____ pounds.

5. Divide this difference by your desired weight to determine the percentage you are overweight or underweight.

   Percentage overweight or underweight (indicate with + or −) _____ %.

Method for determination of desirable weight

The following method, presented by Willoughby,[20] provides a good measure of what the optimal weight should be, taking into account various body-segment widths and diameters.

Six measurements are necessary for both men and women (each is made to the nearest half inch).

Fig. 8-10. Determination of shoulder width.

1. *Shoulder width* (use wooden calipers and measure from the tip of the acromial process to the tip of the acromial process on the other side) (Fig. 8-10).

   Shoulder width = _____ inches.

2. *Iliac width* (use wooden calipers and measure from iliac crest to iliac crest) (Fig. 8-11).

   Iliac width = _____ inches.

3. *Hip width* (use wooden calipers and measure from the most lateral point on each side of the upper part of the femur) (Fig. 8-12).

   Hip width = _____ inches.

4. *Wrist girth* (use tape measure and include the bony knob).

   Wrist girth = _____ inches.

5. *Knee girth* (use tape measure and measure at the middle of the patella).

   Knee girth = _____ inches.

6. *Ankle girth* (use tape measure and measure at the *smallest* point—do not include the bony knob).

   Ankle girth = _____ inches.

The following calculations are necessary:

For women

$0.59 \times$ Shoulder width = _____
$0.75 \times$ Iliac width   = _____
$1.33 \times$ Hip width   = _____
$2.70 \times$ Wrist girth   = _____
$1.77 \times$ Knee girth   = _____
$3.00 \times$ Ankle girth   = _____
TOTAL   = _____

Corrected ankle girth = Total/12
                      = _____

Fig. 8-11. Determination of iliac width.

Fig. 8-12. Determination of hip width.

For men

0.55 × Shoulder width	=	_____
0.78 × Iliac width	=	_____
1.36 × Hip width	=	_____
2.28 × Wrist girth	=	_____
1.78 × Knee girth	=	_____
3.00 × Ankle girth	=	_____
TOTAL	=	_____

Corrected ankle girth = Total/12

= _____

Table 8-8. Desirable weight per inch of height for men and women

Corrected ankle girth	Desirable body weight per inch of height	
	Women	Men
7.0	1.41	—
7.1	1.45	—
7.2	1.50	—
7.3	1.54	—
7.4	1.58	1.72
7.5	1.62	1.77
7.6	1.67	1.81
7.7	1.71	1.86
7.8	1.75	1.91
7.9	1.80	1.96
8.0	1.85	2.01
8.1	1.89	2.06
8.2	1.94	2.11
8.3	1.99	2.16
8.4	2.04	2.21
8.5	2.08	2.27
8.6	2.13	2.32
8.7	2.18	2.37
8.8	2.23	2.43
8.9	2.28	2.49
9.0	2.34	2.54
9.1	2.39	2.60
9.2	2.44	2.66
9.3	2.50	2.71
9.4	2.54	2.77
9.5	—	2.83
9.6	—	2.89
9.7	—	2.95
9.8	—	3.01
9.9	—	3.07
10.0	—	3.14

The optimal weight per inch of height is now determined by consulting Table 8-8 for the figure that corresponds to your corrected ankle girth.

Multiply your height (inches) by the figure obtained from Table 8-8 to find your desirable weight.

Desirable weight = _____ pounds.

FOODS REQUIRED BY THE BODY

The three basic foodstuffs are fats, proteins, and carbohydrates. During the process of digestion each of these is broken into its simplest form and used as a source of energy or for the production of new tissue.

Protein. Protein is needed primarily to build, repair, and regulate the function of the body's cells. It is found mainly in meat, fish, poultry, eggs, milk, cheese, and bread. Proteins constitute approximately 15% of the average American diet.

Carbohydrate. Carbohydrate is the major source of energy for the body. Carbohydrates make up approximately 45% of the typical American diet and often are referred to as starches and sugars. Foods that are high in carbohydrate content are fruits, bread, milk, and potatoes.

Fat. Fat is a secondary source of energy and makes up about 40% of the average American diet. It is found primarily in butter, margarine, oils, meat, whole milk, chocolate, and nuts. Moderate deposits of fat in the body tissues serve as a reserve fuel supply, and some deposits are necessary for the support and protection of certain vital organs. However, excessive deposits may result in added stress on the heart and joints and can result in decreased functioning of the body.

ENERGY

Energy may be defined as the capacity to perform work. Actually, there are two types of energy: (1) potential—stored energy—and (2) kinetic—active energy. Just as the automobile can convert gasoline to power, so the human body converts potential energy from food into kinetic energy in the form of heat and work.

The Calorie

The common unit of measurement for measuring energy is the kilocalorie, or, as it is commonly known, the Calorie. One Calorie is the amount of heat that is necessary to raise 1 kg of water 1° Celsius. It can be used to express the potential energy of food and the amount of energy used by the body in performing various activities.

Caloric intake

The caloric content of the food ingested can be measured. To determine the number of Calories in any food, the food is dehydrated and burned in a special piece of equipment called a calorimeter. When the food is burned, the in-

crease in temperature is measured, and thus the caloric content of the food is determined. The caloric equivalent for each of the three basic foods is presented in Table 8-9.

It can be seen that if the total amount of carbohydrate, fat, and protein is known, caloric equivalents for various foods can be determined. These have been calculated, and the values for certain selected foods are presented in Table 8-10. A more detailed table may be found in most nutrition books.

Table 8-9. Energy available from the three basic types of food

Type of food	Calories/gram
Carbohydrates	4.0
Fats	9.0
Proteins	4.0

Table 8-10. Caloric values for certain selected foods

Food	Serving	Calories
Apple	1 small	75
Apple pie	1/6	275
Applesauce (can)	½ cup	100
Apricots	5 medium	100
Asparagus	12 stalks	25
Bacon (fried)	3 strips	100
Banana	1	100
Banana split	1	450
Beef Stroganoff	average	350
Blueberry muffin	average	150
Bologna	2 ounces	125
Bouillon	1 cup	25
Bread	1 slice	65
Butter	1 pat	50
Cantaloupe	½	50
Cauliflower	1 cup	30
Cheese (American)	1 slice	100
Cheesecake	1 average	350
Chewing gum	1 stick	6
Chicken (baked)	average	200
Chili	½ cup	175
Chocolate bar	average	100
Chocolate cake	1 average	250

Table 8-10. Caloric values for certain selected foods—cont'd

Food	Serving	Calories
Cinnamon roll	average	100
Clams	12 medium	100
Cocoa (with milk)	1 cup	235
Coffee (black)	1 cup	0
Coffee (with cream)	1 cup	30
Coffee (with cream and sugar)	1 cup	65
Coleslaw	6 ounces	20
Corn (fresh frozen)	1 cup	140
Cornflakes	1 cup	100
Corned beef	4 ounces	250
Cottage cheese	1 cup	215
Crackers, graham	3 medium	75
Crackers, soda	6	100
Cream cheese	1 tablespoon	50
Cupcakes (iced)	1 small	150
Dressing (Italian)	1 tablespoon	50
Dressing (Thousand Island)	1 tablespoon	100
Egg (boiled)	1	75
Egg (scrambled)	1	150
Fish (haddock)	average	180
Fish (tuna)	½ cup	250
Frankfurter	1 average	125
Frankfurter roll	1	125
French toast	1 slice	125
Fudge	1-inch square	110
Ginger ale	6 ounces	75
Grapefruit	½ small	50
Ham (baked)	average	350
Hamburger (broiled)	2 ounces	200
Hot fudge sundae	2 scoops	400
Ice cream (vanilla)	average	150
Ice cream soda	1	350
Jam (strawberry)	1 tablespoon	50
Jello	average	100
Lamb chop	1-inch thick	250
Lemon meringue pie	1 piece	350
Lettuce	¼ head	10
Lobster tail	4 ounces	100
Macaroni and cheese	½ cup	225
Martini	1	125
Meat loaf	average	225
Milk	¾ cup	125
Milk (skimmed)	1 cup	85
Muffins	1 average	125
Nuts (Brazil)	2 average	50
Olives	6 small	50

Food	Serving	Calories
Omelet (cheese)	2 eggs	200
Onion (fried)	1	150
Onion (raw)	1 large	50
Onion soup (French)	8-ounce cup	150
Orange	1 medium	75
Orange juice (can)	4 ounces	70
Pancakes	1 4½-inch diameter	100
Peaches	1 medium	50
Peanut butter	1 tablespoon	100
Pickles (dill)	1 large	15
Pickles (sweet)	1 small	25
Pizza with sausage	⅙ (12-inch diameter)	250
Pork chop	1 medium	225
Potato (baked)	1 medium	125
Potato (mashed)	1	180
Potato (hashed brown)	1 medium	225
Potato (french fried)	6	100
Potato chips	½ cup	100
Pretzels	6	100
Pudding (chocolate)	½ cup	250
Ravioli	1	75
Roast beef	6 ounces	75
Salt	⅛ teaspoon	0
Soup (chicken noodle)	1 cup	125
Sour cream	¼ cup	200
Spaghetti with meat sauce	1 serving	375
Spare ribs	6	250
Steak (porterhouse)	average	400
Steak (T-bone)	average	200
Tomato (fresh)	1 medium	25
Tomato juice	1 cup	50
Turkey	average	175
Waffle	1	225
Water	1 cup	0
Wheat (puffed)	1 ounce	105
Wine (white)	wine glass	135
Yogurt	1 cup	165

Energy expenditure

The energy expenditure of each activity may be calculated by measuring the amount of oxygen used in performing the activity. There is a direct relationship between energy expenditure and oxygen consumption because oxygen is used to burn food in producing the necessary energy. It takes approximately 1 liter of oxygen to burn 5 Calories of food. The amount of oxygen used by the body is obviously an important measurement. For example, if a person exercises so that he uses 4 liters of oxygen per minute, for each minute that he continues to exercise he will use 4 × 5, or 20, Calories—equivalent to 1,200 Calories for each hour that he exercises. This is a very fast rate of work and would correspond to marathon running at a rate of approximately 12 miles per hour. It is therefore possible to have a subject perform an activity for a given time and to measure the amount of oxygen that is used. This can then be converted to the number of Calories used in performing the task.

The energy expenditure for different tasks will vary according to the person's skill level, body weight, and other factors. However, it is possible to obtain a good approximation of a person's energy expenditure by consulting ta-

Table 8-11. Energy expenditure for certain selected physical activities*

Activity	Cal/min/lb	Activity	Cal/min/lb
Archery	.034	Running	
Badminton		5.5 mph	.071
Moderate	.038	6.0 mph	.080
Vigorous	.065	7.0 mph	.090
Baseball	.030	9.0 mph	.100
Basketball		10.0 mph	.115
Half court	.028	12.0 mph	.130
Moderate	.045	Sailing	.020
Competitive	.066	Skating	
Bicycling		Moderate	.040
Slow (5.5 mph)	.025	Vigorous	.065
Moderate (10 mph)	.050	Skiing	
Fast (13 mph)	.071	Downhill	.060
Bowling	.030	Level (5 mph)	.078
Calisthenics	.033	Snowshoeing (2.5 mph)	.067
Canoeing		Soccer	.063
Slow (2.5 mph)	.023	Squash	.070
Fast (4.0 mph)	.047	Swimming	
Dancing		Crawl stroke at 1 mph	.045
Moderate	.030	(rate 25 yd in 51 sec)	
Vigorous	.045	Crawl stroke at 1.6 mph	.076
Fishing	.016	(rate 25 yd in 31 sec)	
Football	.060	Crawl stroke at 2.2 mph	.176
Golf	.036	(rate 25 yd in 23 sec)	
Gymnastics		Recreational	.038
Light	.022	Table tennis	.030
Heavy	.056	Tennis	.040
Handball	.065	Volleyball	.030
Hiking	.065	Walking	
Hill climbing	.060	2 mph	.020
Judo and karate	.087	3.5 mph	.031
Paddleball	.066	4.5 mph	.082
Pool	.025	In 12-18 inches snow	.082
		Water skiing	.053
		Wrestling	.053

*Values are adapted from a number of different sources, including references 12, 13, 15, and 18.

bles prepared from actual measurements. The energy expenditure figures for certain selected activities are given in Table 8-11.

It should be stressed that these are average figures and will vary according to skill level. The difference attributable to weight can be determined by taking the Calories per minute per pound and multiplying by the number of pounds that the person weighs and the number of minutes that the activity is performed. For example, if a person weighing 200 pounds ran at 5 miles per hour for 30 minutes, he would use 0.050 × 30 × 200, or 300 Calories for that half hour.

Energy balance

Regardless of whether a person tries to control weight by diet or by exercise, it is the balance between food intake and energy expenditure that will determine whether the program will be successful or not.

A neutral energy balance exists when the caloric intake is equal to the caloric expenditure (Fig. 8-13, *A*). Under these conditions the body weight should remain constant and should nei-

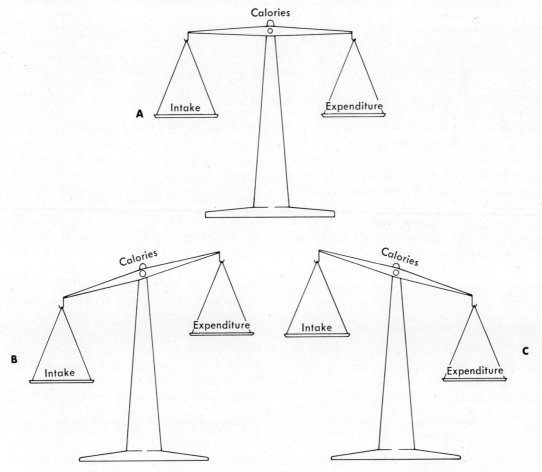

Fig. 8-13. A, Neutral energy balance, in which caloric intake and caloric expenditure are balanced. **B,** Positive energy balance, in which the caloric intake is greater than the caloric expenditure. **C,** Negative energy balance, in which the caloric expenditure is greater than the caloric intake.

Table 8-12. Energy expenditure for everyday tasks*

Everyday tasks	Cal/min/lb	Everyday tasks	Cal/min/lb
Sleeping	.008	Standing, light activity	.016
Lying quietly	.009	House painting	.023
Sitting, eating	.011	Sweeping floors	.024
Mental work, seated	.011	Dressing and showering	.024
Sitting	.011	Carpenter work	.025
Standing	.012	Making bed	.027
Conversing	.012	Cleaning windows	.028
Sitting writing	.012	Ironing	.028
Washing dishes	.012	Farming and planting	.031
Cooking	.013	Gardening	.032
Lecturing	.014	Pick and shovel work	.043
Driving a car	.015	Shoveling sand	.044
Office work	.016	Chopping wood	.049
Light housework	.016		

*Values are adapted from a number of different sources including references 12, 13, 15, and 18.

ther increase nor decrease by any appreciable amount.

A positive energy balance exists when the caloric intake is greater than the caloric expenditure (Fig. 8-13, *B*). The excess food is stored in the form of fat, and the body weight will increase.

In a negative energy balance situation, the opposite is true. The number of Calories used will be greater than the number of Calories consumed (Fig. 8-13, *C*). The extra energy is supplied by the burning of fat, and the body fat and weight will be reduced.

Caloric equivalent of one pound of fat

A few simple calculations make it possible to determine how many Calories are the equivalent of 1 pound of fat. The following information is known:

$$1 \text{ gram of fat} = 9 \text{ Calories}$$
$$1 \text{ pound of fat} = 453 \text{ g}$$

Thus the caloric equivalent of 1 pound of fat is 453 × 9, or 4,077 Calories.

If a person takes in 4,000 Calories a day and uses only 3,000, then each day he takes in ap-

proximately 1,000 Calories more than he uses. Obviously, for each four days that this situation exists he will accumulate an excess of 4,000 Calories, which is approximately equivalent to 1 pound of fat.

Determination of caloric intake

For an individual to obtain a good indication of his caloric intake, he should select a typical weekday and a typical day of the weekend. He should record carefully everything consumed on these days and convert that to Calories by consulting a table of caloric food values. For a more accurate indication of caloric intake, determinations should be made for several such days. The data obtained should be presented on p. 103. If a more accurate indication is desired, both the caloric intake and caloric expenditure should be kept over several days.

Determination of caloric expenditure

For an individual to obtain a good indication of his caloric expenditure, he should estimate the time spent at different activities for the same two days used for the caloric intake. The energy expenditure listing in Table 8-12 should be con-

Table 8-13. Determination of energy balance

	Day 1	Day 2
Total Calories expended		
Total caloric intake		
Difference		
Energy balance (positive or negative)		
Estimated number of pounds you should lose/gain during one year*		

*One pound of fat = 4,000 Calories.

sulted to determine the number of Calories involved. These data should be recorded on p. 102.

The obtained results should be summarized in Table 8-13 and determination made, on this basis, of how the weight should be adjusted.

WEIGHT CONTROL
Exercise as a means of controlling weight

Many persons who are genuinely concerned with losing excess weight have concentrated only on counting the number of Calories in their diets and have completely neglected the role that increased activity can play. For those who are overweight, increasing the amount of physical activity can be just as important as decreasing the food intake. A sensible approach involves a dietary restriction with a progressive buildup of exercise. By simply reducing food intake by 400 Calories per day, it will take 10 days to lose a pound of fat if the activity level remains constant. However, if the activity level is increased by playing an hour of tennis per day or walking an additional hour per day, then it may take just 5 days to lose the pound of fat.

Several studies have indicated that lack of exercise is the most important cause of the "creeping" obesity found in modern mechanized society. Rony,[18] for example, suggests that laziness, or a decreased tendency toward muscular activity, is a primary characteristic of obese children. He was able to show that they avoided unnecessary activity, outdoor play, and athletics. In a similar study, Bronstein et al.[2] found that most of the 35 obese children who were studied spent most of their leisure time in sedentary activities. Green[5] studied more than 200 overweight adult patients in whom the beginning of obesity could be traced directly to a sudden decrease in activity.

When one considers that few occupations now require vigorous physical activity, it is understandable that a large percentage of the adult population is considered overweight. For although there is more time available for recreation, few people use this time in activities that give them exercise.

Misconceptions concerning weight control

Until recent years the role of exercise in weight control programs has been minimized. The reason for this appears to be that many persons lack sufficient information concerning the relationship between exercise and weight control. Also two basic *misconceptions* relating to the role of exercise in weight control have been widely held. Mayer summarizes these as follows:

1. Exercise requires relatively little caloric expenditure and, therefore, increased physical activity hardly changes the caloric balance.

2. An increase in physical activity is always automatically followed by an increase in appetite and food intake and may, therefore, actually impair the success of the weight control program.[12]

Scientific evidence relating to these statements clearly shows that both of them are false.[7]

Energy expenditure in exercise

The average adult man will use from 2,400 to 4,500 Calories a day, depending on the level of activity. Persons who are very active, such as laborers and athletes, may require as many as 6,000 Calories per day—a fact that has been known for many years. Johnson[7] has shown that when a group of university students increased their caloric intake from 3,000 to 6,000 Calories per day, they were able to maintain a constant weight by increasing the amount of exercise in which they participated each day.

It was shown previously that 1 pound of fat is equivalent to approximately 4,000 Calories. The caloric expenditure for certain tasks also was presented. It is possible therefore to calculate the number of hours that must be spent participating in an activity to lose 1 pound of fat. These figures are presented in Table 8-14 for certain selected activities.

This information suggests that losing weight through exercise would be difficult. For example, one would have to play volleyball for 17 hours to lose 1 pound of fat. This is equivalent to 10.9 hours of golf or 8.5 hours of tennis. The fact that has been overlooked, however, is that

the activity does not have to be performed continuously. One must look at the "long haul" concept of weight control. If a person plays tennis for 1 hour a day, 4 days a week, over a period of a year, this will account for approximately 25 pounds. This emphasizes one point: for exercise to be beneficial it must be performed regularly. Another point is important. If a person walked an extra mile a day instead of riding, this would account for a loss of almost 30 pounds over a period of a year, provided his caloric intake remained constant. This is really not an impractical amount of time to spend, and if it is desirable to lose weight faster or to lose more weight, it simply becomes necessary to increase the amount of activity.

Food intake and exercise

The claim that an increase in physical activity always causes an increase in appetite and food intake that equals or is greater in energy value than the energy cost of the exercise also is false. Laboratory tests using rats have shown that when the amount of exercise performed is moderate, from 20 minutes to 1 hour, the food intake does not increase—in fact, it actually shows a decrease. These results are presented in Fig. 8-14. Not only was there a decrease in the

Table 8-14. Caloric expenditure and weight control for certain activities for a 170-pound man

Activity	Cal/hr	Hours to lose 1 pound of fat
Walking	337	11.8
Basketball	479	8.4
Volleyball	235	17.0
Golf	367	10.9
Tennis	469	8.5
Wrestling	950	4.2

Fig. 8-14. Relationship between food intake, energy expenditure, and body weight. (Adapted from Mayer.[11])

daily caloric intake, but there was also a decrease in body weight. With long periods of sustained activity the food intake did increase, but the weight remained constant at this optimal level, since the extra activity balanced out the extra caloric intake.

Mayer[11] also was able to obtain similar results working with adults. This study was conducted in India, where it was possible to control adequately many relevant factors. The results of this study are presented in Fig. 8-15. These results indicate that light and medium work result in a decrease in caloric intake and in body weight and that heavy and very heavy work result in an increase in caloric intake, but body weight remained constant.

It was emphasized previously that the start of obesity for many persons has been associated with a decline in activity. Professional or college athletes in training usually have very little trouble maintaining their weight, despite the fact that they usually eat all the food that they want to. Yet many athletes do not maintain their activity level or do not decrease their food intake when they retire and so experience a prob-

lem controlling their weight. This is a problem also encountered by many individuals when they finish school and go to work. If their job is sedentary or inactive, they tend to exercise less but continue to eat as much as ever. The result, of course, is that they increase their weight very rapidly.

Johnson, Burke, and Mayer[6] compared systematically the caloric intake and activity level in carefully paired groups of obese and normal-weight school girls. The time spent by the obese girls participating in any type of exercise was less than half that spent by the nonobese girls. The remaining time spent by the obese group was used for "nonactive" activities. The caloric intake was higher in the nonobese group than in the obese group.

Cristakis[4] presents information showing how many minutes of certain selected activities are necessary to "balance out" the caloric value of certain common foods. A partial listing of his information is presented in Table 8-15. The numbers in the activity columns refer to the number of minutes that the activity must be performed to "balance out" the caloric content of

Fig. 8-15. Body weight and caloric intake as related to physical activity in man. (Adapted from Mayer.[11])

each serving of food. For example, one large apple contains 101 Calories. This table indicates that to use an equivalent number of Calories one would either have to read for 56 minutes, bowl for 23 minutes, play golf for 20 minutes, walk for 20 minutes, play tennis for 14 minutes, or sleep for 87 minutes. The figures contained in this table are applicable to a person weighing 150 pounds.

The part that exercise can play in weight control is summarized in Fig. 8-16, which demonstrates very clearly the fact that activity burns

up extra Calories that would otherwise be stored as excess fat in the body. The more vigorous the activity, the more Calories are used up. It is important to realize, however, that activity does not have to be continuous to result in a loss in weight. The total amount of work will determine the number of Calories used.

Diet as a means to weight control

Most of the American adult population rely solely on various diets as a means to weight control. Each week new diets are introduced

Table 8-15. Balance between caloric intake of selected foods and caloric expenditure of selected activities

Type of food	Calories per serving	Minutes required for expenditure					
		Reading	Bowling	Golf	Walking	Tennis	Sleeping
Large apple	101	56	23	20	20	14	87
Boiled egg	77	43	17	15	15	11	66
Bread and butter	78	43	18	16	16	11	67
Two strips bacon	96	53	22	19	19	14	82
One glass beer	114	63	26	23	23	16	98
One glass milk	166	92	38	33	32	33	142
Cheese pizza	180	100	41	36	35	25	154
T-bone steak	235	131	53	47	45	33	201
Hamburger	350	194	80	70	67	49	300
Strawberry shortcake	400	222	91	80	77	56	343

Fig. 8-16. Relationship between exercise, food intake, and accumulation of body fat. Either of the above two situations may apply to each individual. In each case the large circle represents the total caloric intake. It can be seen that if the excess energy is not used by participation in regular exercise, excess fat will accumulate. (Drawing by Eugene Sinervo; adapted from Royal Canadian Air Force Physical Fitness Program.)

that guarantee one will lose a certain amount of weight or a given number of inches from various areas of the body. Research has shown that more than 9.5 million Americans are on diets at any given time during the year, whereas an additional 16.4 million indicate that they are watching their weight. A further 26.1 million indicate that they are ''concerned'' about their waistlines.[22]

In the same article the following summary of the effects of diet on weight control is presented:

The 79 million American adults who are overweight today have more than their excess pounds in common. One central fact of their lives is that many millions of them will soon be going on yet another remarkable new diet. Chances are that this regimen will offer to relieve the duties of the burden of counting Calories. It will not cause hunger pangs. It will enable its adherents to lose precisely as many unsightly pounds as they choose. Unhappily, this promising new diet will be just that: promising. It may turn out to be damaging to the dieter's health, and it is practically guaranteed not to have any lasting effect on his or her overweight problem.[22]

Evidence is available to show that diets are successful with only a small percentage of persons. One study showed that out of every 100 who were concerned enough about weight control to see their doctor, only 7% actually attained their desired weight and only 2% were able to maintain this for a period of 1 year. Diets are not very successful because they cause an imbalance in the food intake. For example, a low carbohydrate diet may contain as much as 70% of daily Calories from fats. Apart from being damaging to a person's health, eating the same kinds of food each day becomes monotonous; as a result, most people do not maintain a diet for more than 1 or 2 months. Usually, once they go off the diet, they put the weight back on again quickly.

What is necessary for weight control is a permanent change in daily eating habits, so that a person's caloric intake is reduced and the caloric expenditure increased until a negative energy balance is established.

In summary, the following can be said as to the effects of diets:

1. Diets are a successful means of controlling weight for only a small percentage of persons.
2. Certain diets may result in a reduction in weight but at the same time may be damaging to one's health.
3. Most diets create an imbalance in the food intake, and therefore few individuals adhere to them for any length of time.
4. There are few new diets.
5. A diet will be successful only if a negative energy balance exists within the body.

Exercise versus diet as a means of weight control

A popular belief is that dieting is a more successful way of controlling weight than exercise. This belief is based on the premise that it is easier to reduce caloric intake than to increase caloric expenditure.

When the effects of exercise and diet on body composition are compared, the results are interesting. A study by Oscai and Holloszy using rats showed that after 18 weeks of either food restriction or exercise, exercise resulted in a greater reduction in fat. With dieting, a large proportion of the weight loss was from water loss.[14]

In two separate studies[9,23] involving human subjects, similar results were obtained. Both studies concluded that exercise is superior to diet in reducing body fat. Diet or caloric restriction does result in loss of weight; however, this loss if achieved primarily by loss of protein and water.

Exercise and diet can be combined to achieve the quickest and most effective way to reduce weight and body fat. The success of a good weight-reducing program will depend on the total amount of work performed. Running or walking 2 miles per day will result in minimal reduction compared to running or walking 6 miles per day. The continuity and intensity of the activity are insignificant factors in weight control.

Suggestions to follow when attempting to lose weight

1. A proper diet must provide all the necessary nutrients in sufficient amounts.
2. The maximum weight loss rate should be 2 pounds per week.
3. A caloric intake of fewer than 1500 Calories/day for men and 1200 Calories/day for women is poorly tolerated over long periods of time.
4. By increasing physical activity a person should have a deficit of 500 to 1200 Calories per day without reducing caloric intake below the above limit.
5. The total percentage of fat Calories in the diet should be reduced to 30% to 35% (from 40% to 50%), with the level of saturated fatty acids less than 10% of the total Calories.
6. A balanced diet containing no less than 12% to 14% protein, no more than 30% to 35% fats, and the remaining percentages from carbohydrates is best if it is made up of foods of sufficient variety.

SUMMARY

Basically, exercise does not use a large number of Calories. A 10- to 15-minute exercise program may use only 140 to 200 Calories. Comparing this to the caloric value of a slice of bread—75 Calories—or a piece of pie—250 Calories—one can see that a very small amount of food is the equivalent of a considerable amount of exercise. Those who exercise regularly should not be lulled into believing that if they are exercising 30 minutes a day, they can eat as much as they wish.

An individual certainly can use additional Calories by increasing his daily physical activity level, by climbing three flights of stairs four times a day rather than riding the elevator, by walking instead of riding, and by taking time to exercise regularly. The important point is that a man with a daily expenditure of 3,000 Calories will slowly lose weight if he takes in fewer than 3,000 Calories a day and will gain weight if he eats more than 3,000 Calories per day. Because a pound of fat is the equivalent of about 4,000 Calories, changes in caloric intake or caloric expenditure do not usually result in *rapid* weight fluctuations. Significant changes in weight are a result of a more prolonged reduction in food, together with an increase in caloric expenditure. Mayer summarizes the situation as follows:

Inactivity is the most important factor explaining the frequency of "creeping" overweight in modern Western societies. The regulation of food intake was never designed to adapt to the highly mechanized sedentary conditions of modern life. Adaptation to these conditions without development of obesity means that either the individual will have to step up his activity or that he will be mildly or acutely hungry all his life. The first alternative is difficult, especially as present conditions in the United States offer little inducement to walking and are often poorly organized as regards facilities for adult exercise. But if the first alternative of stepping up activity is difficult, it is well to remember that the second alternative, lifetime hunger, is so much more difficult to rely on.[12]

Diet alone is a much slower method for reducing weight than if combined with a good exercise program. It should be remembered that this method of relying only on a diet is successful with only a small percentage of persons and that many of these diets create an imbalance in food intake that may be quite hazardous to the individual's health.

REFERENCES

1. Allsen, P. E., Harrison, J. M., and Vance, B.: Fitness for life: an individualized approach, Dubuque, Iowa, 1975, Wm. C. Brown Company, Publishers.
2. Bronstein, I. P., et al.: Obesity in childhood, American Journal of Diseases of Children **63:**238, 1942.

3. Brozek, J., and Keys, A.: Relative body weight, age, and fatness, Geriatrics **8**:70, 1953.

4. Christakis, G.: An anti-coronary club for prudent men. In The healthy life, New York, 1966, Time, Inc., p. 76.

5. Green, J. A.: Clinical studies of the etiology of obesity, American Internal Medicine **12**:1797, 1939.

6. Johnson, M. L., Burke, B. S., and Mayer, J.: Caloric intake in relation to energy output, American Journal of Clinical Nutrition **4**:231, 1956.

7. Johnson, R. E.: Exercise and weight control, a statement prepared for the committee on Exercise and Physical Fitness of the American Medical Association and the President's Council of Physical Fitness, Urbana, Aug., 1967, University of Illinois.

8. Johnston, F. E., Hamill, D. V., and Lemeshaw, S.: Skinfold thickness in youths 12-17 years of age, U.S. National Center for Health Statistics II, No. 132, Washington, D.C., 1974, Department of Health, Education, and Welfare.

9. Kenrick, M. M., Bull, M. F., and Canary, T. J.: Exercise and fat loss in obese patients, Proceedings of annual meeting of American Academy of Physical Medicine and Rehabilitation, San Juan, P.R., 1972.

10. Land of the fat, Time magazine, **111**:53, Jan. 2, 1978.

11. Mayer, J.: Obesity diagnosis, Postgraduate Medicine **25**:469, 1959.

12. Mayer, J.: Overweight: causes, cost, and control, Englewood Cliffs, N.J., 1968, Prentice-Hall, Inc.

13. Melograno, V., and Klinzing, J. E.: An orientation to total fitness, Dubuque, Iowa, 1974, Kendall/Hunt Publishing Company, p. 127.

14. Oscai, L. B., and Holloszy, J. O.: Effects of weight changes produced by exercise, food restriction or overeating on body composition, Journal of Clinical Investigation **48**:2124-2128, 1969.

15. Overweight: its significance and prevention, New York, 1963, Metropolitan Life Insurance Co., p. 31.

16. Pollock, M., et al.: Prediction of body density in young and middle-aged men, Journal of Applied Physiology **40**:300, March, 1976.

17. Pollock, M., et al.: Prediction of body density in young and middle-aged women, Journal of Applied Physiology **39**:745, April, 1975.

18. Rony, H. R.: Obesity and leanness, Philadelphia, 1940, Lea & Febiger.

19. Sinning, W.: Use and misuse of anthropometric estimates of body composition, Journal of Health, Physical Education, and Recreation, Feb., 1980, p. 43.

20. Willoughby, D. P.: An anthropometric method for arriving at the optimal proportions of the body in the adult individual, Research Quarterly **3**:48, 1932.

21. Wilmore, J., and Behnke, A. R.: An anthropometric estimation of body density and lean body weight in young women, American Journal of Clinical Nutrition **23**:267-274, 1970.

22. Wyden, P., and Wyden, B.: Why diet and exercise fads won't turn your fatness into fitness. In The healthy life, New York, 1966, Time, Inc.

23. Zuti, W. B., and Golding, L.: Comparing diet and exercise as weight reduction tools, The Physician and Sports Medicine **4**:59-62, 1976.

Name _____

Day and hour laboratory section meets _____

Laboratory instructor _____

Date _____

DAILY CALORIC EXPENDITURE

Date _____

Day 1 (weekday) Body weight _____			Date _____	Day 2 (weekend) Body weight _____		
Activity	Minutes of par- ticipation	Cal/min/lb	Calories expended*	Activity	Minutes of par- ticipation	Cal/min/lb	Calories expended*
Total Calories used per day _____				Total Calories used per day _____			

*To calculate this, multiply cal/min/lb by the number of minutes of participation and then by your body weight.

Name _____

Day and hour laboratory section meets _____

Laboratory instructor _____

Date _____

DAILY CALORIC INTAKE

Date _____ Body weight _____

Day 1 (weekday)

Time of day	Type of food	Amount	Calories

Total Calories consumed per day _____

Date _____ Body weight _____

Day 2 (weekend)

Time of day	Type of food	Amount	Calories

Total Calories consumed per day _____

Fill in totals on following page.

Name _____ **Date** _____

Day and hour laboratory section meets _____

Laboratory instructor _____

SUMMARY SHEET FOR OVERWEIGHT AND BODY FAT EVALUATION

Height _____ inches   Weight _____ pounds

Percentage body fat _____   Percentage overweight (height-weight charts) _____

Desirable weight (Willoughby method) _____

Calculated energy balance (positive or negative) _____

Average caloric expenditure (average of day 1 and day 2) _____

Average caloric intake (average of day 1 and day 2) _____

Skinfold measurements (mm)

    Chest (men only) _____

    Subscapular   _____

    Thigh   _____

    Suprailiac   _____

    Abdominal   _____

    Triceps   _____

    Midaxillary   _____

CHAPTER 9

Exercise and health

What do you know about exercise and health?

T F

☐ ☐ **1.** Many diseases are attributable to lack of sufficient activity.

☐ ☐ **2.** The benefits of exercise are permanent.

☐ ☐ **3.** Without sufficient activity the body begins to deteriorate and possibly becomes more susceptible to certain illnesses and disease.

☐ ☐ **4.** Training decreases the oxygen requirement for work.

☐ ☐ **5.** Regular exercise has been shown to reduce the resting heart rate.

☐ ☐ **6.** If a trained and an untrained subject perform the same work task, the trained person will exhibit a higher heart rate.

☐ ☐ **7.** People who have desk jobs are more susceptible to low back pain than active workers.

☐ ☐ **8.** Low back pain is often the result of muscular deficiency.

☐ ☐ **9.** Physically active people are able to recover from a heart attack more frequently than sedentary people because collateral circulation is better developed.

☐ ☐ **10.** Exercise may reduce the free fatty acids and other lipids circulating in the blood.

PERSONAL BENEFITS OF REGULAR EXERCISE

Most people want to know why they should exercise regularly and what benefits they can derive from regular participation in a well-designed exercise program.

In order to evaluate the benefits of exercise it is important to identify the reasons people first become involved in exercise. The results from a recent national survey are summarized in Table 9-1.[10]

The degree of success achieved by participants in organized exercise programs obviously depends on the frequency of participation. The percentages of reported beneficial effects, both

Table 9-1. Reasons for becoming involved in regular exercise

Reason	Percentage of respondents
To feel better in general	51
To stay healthy	45
To lose weight	41
For recreation and enjoyment	37
To increase strength	36
To become fit	33
To become more healthy	24
To strengthen the heart and lungs	24
Doctor recommended it	17
To socialize and meet new friends	8
Other	4

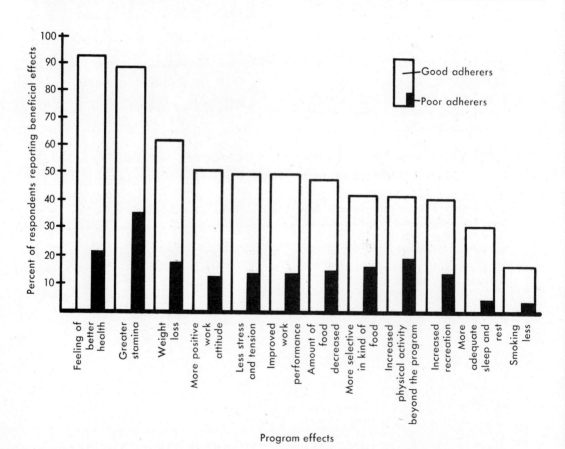

Fig. 9-1. Exercise program effects as they relate to participation. (From Dunbeck et al.[5])

for those who participated regularly in an exercise program and for those who did not, are compared in Fig. 9-1.

For the average person there are many benefits associated with regular physical activity[8]; some of these are summarized in Table 9-2.

Changes that occur as a result of participation in an exercise program can be measured precisely. Such changes are reported in a recent study summarized in Table 9-3.[1]

Similar results have been obtained for 84 new participants enrolled in the adult physical fitness programs at Northern Michigan University during 1978 and 1979. An individualized aerobic exercise program was designed for each person in this program with participation 3 to 4 days per week for 12 weeks. A summary of these results is presented in Table 9-4.

The percentage changes obtained in any program will be dependent upon the intensity and duration of exercise program. However, a comparison of the two sets of data shows fairly consistent results for these two separate programs.

The data in Table 9-4 indicate an increase in the efficiency of the lungs that allows them to process more air, thus creating an increase in the maximal amount of oxygen that the body is able to utilize. These, of course, result in a corresponding increase in the maximal amount of work that can be performed.

Fig. 9-2. A, Position of the hamstring muscle group in relation to the bone structure when in a sitting posture. If much of the time is spent sitting, this muscle group may become much shorter than it should be. **B,** Effect that a shortening of the hamstring muscles has on the pelvis, when one assumes an upright standing position. (Drawings by Eugene Sinervo; adapted from Johnson et al.[11])

Table 9-2. General health benefits associated with regular physical activity[4]

Major health benefit	Associated factors
Improved health and well-being	Feeling of better health
	More energy available to perform daily tasks
	Increased ability to meet emergencies
	Increased general vitality
Reduced mental and emotional stress	Reduced tension
	Able to relax more
	More adequate sleep and rest
	More positive work attitude
Improved personal appearance	Reduced body weight
	Decreased body fat
	Enhanced self-concept and body image
	Delay of aging process
	Decreased amount of food
	More selective in type of food
	Improved posture and appearance
Decreased incidence of degenerative disease and common health components	Less chance of heart attack
	Greater chance of surviving a heart attack
	Improved fat metabolism
	Decreased levels of cholesterol and triglycerides
	Decreased blood pressure
Improved cardiovascular endurance	Increased musculature of the heart so it can contract more forceably
	Decreased resting heart rate
	Increased stroke volume
	Ability to perform more work before becoming fatigued
	Ability to recover faster following a strenuous task
	Less stress placed on heart during the performance of a submaximal task
	Increased physical work capacity
Improved strength and muscular endurance	Less chance of muscle or joint injury
	Reduction of low back pain problems
	Increased muscle tone
Increase in flexibility	Decreased incidence of low back pain

Table 9-3. Changes in important physiological variables as a result of participation in a regular exercise program

Variable	Pretest score	Posttest score	Percentage change
Resting heart rate	73 beats/min	63 beats/min	14% decrease
Resting blood pressure	133/89	125/77	6%/13% decrease
Cholesterol	240 mg/100 ml	217 mg/100 ml	10% decrease
Percent body fat	21	17	19% decrease
Maximal oxygen consumption (per minute)	28.5 ml/kg body weight	35 ml/kg body weight	23% increase

Table 9-4. Summary of changes in physical fitness variables obtained at Northern Michigan University*

Variable	Pretest		Posttest		Percentage change
	Mean	SD	Mean	SD	
Resting heart rate (beats/min)	76.5	10.9	71.47	11.1	6% decrease
Resting blood pressure (mm Hg)	130/81	18/9	122/78	16/9	6%/4% decrease
Body weight (lb)	172.5	41.0	165.5	40.8	4% decrease
Maximal ventilation (liters)	59.3	17.6	78.8	20.4	32% increase
Maximal oxygen consumption (ml/kg body weight/min)	26.4	7.4	34.0	8.9	29% increase

*N = 84.

CHANGES OCCURRING IN THE BODY RELATING TO CARDIOVASCULAR DISEASE

Several changes take place as a result of regular exercise that could explain why there is a reduction in the incidence of cardiovascular disease for those persons who exercise regularly. These changes include the following:

1. Increase in the efficiency of the heart.
2. Development of collateral circulation in heart.[6]
3. Decreased resting heart rate, meaning more rest for the heart.
4. Quicker clearing of fats from the bloodstream.[3]
5. Decrease in cholesterol and triglycerides.[1]
6. Increased level of high density lipoprotein.[9]
7. Reduction of excess weight and body fat.
8. Decreased blood pressure.

Each of these changes is a possible explanation why regular exercise might reduce the chances of suffering from some form of cardiovascular disease.

EXERCISE AND LOW BACK PAIN

Low back pain is one of the most common complaints among adults in the United States today. It results in many lost hours of work and much discomfort.

Kraus and Raab[13] have classified low back pain as a hypokinetic disease, which they define as a disease caused by insufficient activity. This is in agreement with Feffer,[7] a well-known orthopedic surgeon, who states that "the increase in the incidence of low back pain is related to the increasingly sedentary life we lead. We simply do not get enough exercise."

Low back pain is a "disease" that occurs fairly early in life and appears to be most prevalent from 25 to 35 years of age.

Causes of low back pain

The major cause of low back pain is improper muscular development. The development and maintenance of muscle function is dependent upon its use. The strength of a muscle is directly related to the amount of work that it does. As a muscle works against a resistance, the strength of that muscle will increase. If the muscle does not perform any work, a loss of strength will result. In an inactive person many of the large muscle groups are not used frequently enough. They therefore lack sufficient strength to maintain the correct body alignment, which is one of their specific tasks.

Poor abdominal development is one of the most common causes of low back pain. The pelvis should be tipped up in the front, but if the abdominal muscles are weak, they are unable to exert sufficient pressure to keep the pelvis in place, and it drops down in the front, causing a forward pelvis tilt. This in turn causes the vertebrae in the lower back region to be slightly displaced, and their articular processes press against one another, causing the ache in the lower area of the back.[2]

Another group of muscles associated with low back pain is commonly referred to as the *hamstring muscle group*. This group consists of three muscles—the *biceps femoris,* the *semimembranosus,* and the *semitendinosus* muscles. All three of these muscles lie along the posterior aspect of the thigh and all are associated with movement at both the hip and the knee joints.

The difficulty experienced by most persons in touching the toes with the fingertips without bending the knees is caused by the fact that the hamstring muscles often are not long enough to permit such extreme stretching.[13] This shortening of the hamstring muscle group will often occur in those who spend a large amount of time in a sitting position (Fig. 9-2). If these muscles are not given any stretching exercises, and if they are constantly held in positions that tend to shorten them, they become adjusted to this position. When a person assumes the standing position, both the knee and hip joints are fully extended (Fig. 9-2, *B*). If the hamstring muscles are shorter than they should be, this will cause both direct pain in the immediate area of the muscles and referred pain in the lower back region. Kraus and Raab state that:

In our civilized cities we lead the lives of caged animals. We have no opportunity to move, no chance to respond to outside irritations. Besides, most of us are burdened by emotional problems, adding to the need for release. Since our civilization does not permit the natural responses of fight or flight, and since we do not have vicarious outlets by heavy exercise, tension is stored up in our muscles. This constant tension shortens the muscles and deprives them of elasticity. Once this muscle tightness has reached a sufficiently high level, and lack of physical activity has weakened our tense muscles, the stage is set for the first episode of back pain.[13]

Fig. 9-3. Causes of low back pain. Note that over 80% of low back pain is due to muscular deficiency. (Adapted from Kraus and Raab.[12])

Kraus and Raab present evidence indicating that over 80% of low back pain is caused by muscular deficiency. Their results are summarized in Fig. 9-3. The test used to evaluate these patients was the Kraus-Weber test, which is a test of *minimal* strength and flexibility.[12]

Kraus-Weber test

The Kraus-Weber test is a simple six-item test that can be used effectively to identify individuals who are likely to suffer from low back pain in the future. It should be stressed that this test measures only minimal muscular strength and flexibility. Following is a description of each of the six items that make up this test.

1. *Straight-leg sit-up.* The subject assumes a supine position (faceup) on the floor with hands held behind the neck. With legs straight and feet held down, he simply rolls up into a sitting position, keeping his hands behind his neck. This is a test for minimal strength of the abdominal muscles and also the psoas major muscle.
2. *Bent-leg sit-up.* The subject assumes a supine position on the floor with hands held behind the neck, knees bent, and bottoms of the feet flat on the floor. With feet held down and hands remaining behind the neck, he again rolls up into a sit-

ting position. This is a test for minimal strength of the abdominal muscles.

3. *Forward leg lift.* The subject assumes a supine position on the floor with hands held behind the neck and legs extended. With legs straight, the feet are lifted 10 inches off the floor, and this position is held for 10 seconds. This test is designed to measure minimal strength of the lower abdominal muscles.

4. *Trunk lift.* The subject assumes a prone position (facedown) on the floor, with a pillow under his abdomen. With hands behind the neck and feet and hips held down, the subject raises his trunk and holds this position for 10 seconds. This is a test of minimal strength of the upper back muscles.

5. *Backward leg raise.* Ths subject again assumes a prone position over a pillow. With back and hips held, he must lift his legs and hold them off the ground for 10 seconds. This is a test of minimal strength of the lower back muscles.

6. *Toe touch.* The subject stands erect with legs straight and feet held together. He then reaches down slowly without forcing unnecessarily and touches the floor with his fingers. This position is maintained for a period of 3 seconds. No jerking movements are allowed, and the legs must remain perfectly straight throughout. This is a test of the length of the hamstring muscle group.

Each student is evaluated on each of these items simply on a pass-fail basis. If a person cannot pass all six, he has failed the test. This classifies him as a potential sufferer of low back pain. This is the test that was given to a group of American and European children in 1952. More than 57% of the American children failed to pass one or more of the six items that make up this test. This could partly explain the high incidence of low back pain in this country today.

SUMMARY

The changes outlined in this chapter make it possible for a person to live a fuller and more productive life. An individual is able to perform more work before becoming fatigued or to perform the same amount of work with less physio-

logical stress. Williams[14] summarizes the effects of training as follows: "The objective of training is to permit the performance of an activity with less disturbance to the internal environment and also to increase the activity potential of the individual."

In the discussion on physical fitness, it was indicated that a certain "minimal" level of muscular strength is necessary. Those persons who are unable to manage their own weight and to maintain adequate posture do not possess this "minimal" level of strength. Not meeting this level should indicate that the amount of physical activity of that individual is not sufficient to meet his demands.

Those persons who are potential candidates for low back pain are easy to identify. These individuals should include in their activity programs exercises that will reduce the likelihood of suffering from low back pain. Much time and money could be saved if they would take time to exercise regularly to alleviate low back pain, rather than trying to find alternate, easy, shortcut methods, which really are nonexistent.

REFERENCES

1. Barnes, L.: Selling fitness through health promotion, The Physician and Sports Medicine **8:**119, April, 1980.
2. Brouha, L.: The effect of work on the heart. In Rosenbaum, F. F., and Belknap, E., editors: Work and the heart, New York, 1959, Paul B. Hoeber, Inc., p. 184.
3. Cantone, A.: Physical effort and its effect in reducing alimentary hyperlipemia, Journal of Sports Medicine and Physical Fitness **4:**32, 1964.
4. Corbin, C., et al.: Concepts in physical education, ed. 3, Dubuque, Ia., 1978, Wm. C. Brown, publisher, p. 98.
5. Dunbeck, D. C., et al.: The National Aeronautics and Space Administration—U.S. Public Health Service health evaluation and enhancement, American Journal of Cardiology, Nov. 30, 1972, p. 784.
6. Eckstein, R. W.: Effect of exercise and coronary artery narrowing on coronary collateral circulation, Circulation Research **5:**230, 1957.
7. Feffer, H.: All about backache, Reader's Digest, Dec., 1971, p. 203.
8. Gendel, E. S.: Lack of fitness: a source of chronic ills in women, The Physician and Sports Medicine **6:**85, Feb., 1978.

9. Hartwig, G. H., and Squires, W. G.: Exercise and HDL cholesterol in middle-aged men, The Physician and Sports Medicine **8**:74, Jan., 1980.

10. Health maintenance, Newport Beach, Calif., Nov., 1978, Pacific Mutual Life Insurance Co.

11. Johnson, P. B., et al.: Physical education—a problem-solving approach to health and fitness, New York, 1966, Holt, Rinehart and Winston, Inc.

12. Kraus, H., and Eisenmenger-Weber, S.: Quantitative tabulation of posture evaluation, based on structural and functional measurements, The Physiotherapy Review **26**:235, 1946.

13. Kraus, H., and Raab, W.: Hypokinetic disease, Springfield, Ill., 1961, Charles C Thomas, Publisher, p. 8.

14. Williams, J. G.: Medical aspects of sport and physical fitness, Oxford, 1965, Pergamon Press, p. 12.

CHAPTER 10

Skill and motor ability

What do you know about skill and motor ability?

T F

☐ ☐ **1.** Motor ability and physical fitness are synonymous terms.

☐ ☐ **2.** Football is an activity that should be stressed because it is a good carryover activity.

☐ ☐ **3.** An increased skill level in an activity like handball will be likely to result in an increased heart rate during participation.

☐ ☐ **4.** No activity, regardless of skill level, will be as beneficial as running for the development of cardiovascular endurance.

☐ ☐ **5.** Agility is most important in swimming.

☐ ☐ **6.** The best measure of power is the 50-yard dash.

☐ ☐ **7.** Speed and reaction time are really the same.

☐ ☐ **8.** Athletes are superior to untrained subjects in reaction time.

☐ ☐ **9.** Reaction time is very important in wrestling.

☐ ☐ **10.** Balance may be defined as the ability to maintain the equilibrium of the body.

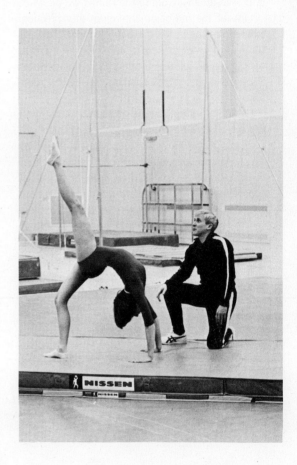

Participation in activities such as basketball, tennis, handball, and swimming can play an important part in the development of physical fitness. For this reason, developing one's skill level in several of these activities is important because the higher the person's skill level is in an activity, the more likely he is to participate in it. We all enjoy doing the things we do well.

One of the major objectives of any physical education program is the development of a person's skill level. A person who performs a skill well is said to exhibit good motor ability. Motor ability can thus be defined as the skillful performance of a physical skill.

Each individual should make an attempt to become skillful in at least one activity and preferably in more than one. The types of activities that a person can enjoy and participate in later in life should be stressed in both high school and college physical education programs. These activities are often referred to as "lifetime" sports and include such activities as bowling, golf, archery, tennis, swimming, hunting, fishing, handball, and paddleball.

In the selection of activities, some thought should be given to whether they can be used later in life and whether they will contribute to the development of physical fitness. Persons usually do not participate in such activities as basketball, baseball, and football later in life, and activities such as archery, volleyball, golf, hunting, and fishing have only minimal, if any, contributions to make toward the development of physical fitness. This is not to say that these are not good recreational activities. However, if a person can select an activity that he enjoys participating in and that will contribute toward the development of physical fitness, it is much better to participate in this activity than in one that can be used only for recreational purposes. The heart rate response to running for 12 minutes at a rate of 9 miles per hour is presented in Fig. 10-1. Also presented is the obtained heart rate for the same subject during participation in racquetball singles competition. It can clearly be seen that both of these activities elevate the heart rate considerably and can be used for the development of physical fitness.

It is also interesting to note that the higher the person's skill level as well as that of his opponent is in a particular sport, the greater energy expenditure is involved. In many instances this

Fig. 10-1. Comparison of heart rate responses for running at 9 mph and participating in one-wall racquetball singles competition.

will result in a greater contribution of these activities to the development of cardiovascular endurance.

COMPONENTS OF MOTOR ABILITY

The six generally recognized components of motor ability are (1) agility, (2) power, (3) coordination, (4) speed, (5) reaction time, and (6) balance.

Agility

Agility may be defined as the ability to change direction accurately and quickly while moving rapidly. In some activities the ability to stop and start and to change direction quickly is much more important than in others. In sports such as basketball, badminton, handball, and tennis, agility is a most important factor. This may be measured by such tasks as the shuttle run and activities that require a quick change of direction.

Probably the most commonly used test for measuring this component is the Illinois Agility Run.[1] The subject assumes a prone position with the hands beside the chest and forehead on the starting line. He jumps up at the starting signal and follows the zigzag pattern shown in Fig. 10-2.

The aim is to complete the pattern in the shortest possible time. Measurement is in terms of seconds and is recorded to the nearest tenth of a second from the starting signal until the subject crosses the finish line. The test must be taken with rubber-soled gym shoes. Two trials are allowed, with at least 2 minutes of rest allowed between them.

The results for the test should be recorded:

Trial 1 _____ seconds

Trial 2 _____ seconds

Best trial _____ seconds

Power

Power is defined as the ability to exert a maximal contraction in one explosive act. It is sometimes referred to as explosive strength. It is dependent on two other factors—strength and speed. A good example of this is the shot put. In this event the participant combines strength and speed as they are coordinated into an explosive movement, with the maximal force being exerted as quickly as possible. The broad jump is another example of an activity in which power is most important. To a lesser degree it is important in the jump shot in basketball. This factor may be measured by the standing broad jump, the medicine ball put, or the jump-and-reach test. No matter what test is used for measuring this factor, the person is required to jump or project himself or some object either as far or as high as possible.[3]

For evaluating power, both the standing broad jump and the jump-and-reach test are

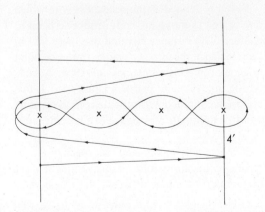

Fig. 10-2. Pattern to be followed for the agility run. Each of the four chairs or cones in the center line are placed 10 feet apart.

good. Because of its ease of administration, the standing broad jump may be preferred over the jump-and-reach test. The standing broad jump measures explosive leg power, which is dependent on speed and strength. A starting line is marked on the floor, and the subject stands with feet apart and toes behind the starting line. He then flexes at the hips, knees, and ankles and, by swinging the arms, jumps as far forward as possible. Measurement is to the nearest inch, from the take-off line to the heel of the foot nearest the take-off line or any portion of the body nearer the line. Two trials are allowed.

The results for the standing broad jump should be recorded:

Trial 1 _____ inches
Trial 2 _____ inches
Best trial _____ inches

Coordination

Coordination can be defined as the integration of separate abilities into the smooth execution of a task. This may involve various parts of the body, such as eye-foot coordination, as in kicking a football, or hand-eye coordination, as in catching a tennis ball. An example might help to demonstrate exactly what is meant by coordination. Consider the breaststroke in swimming. A student can learn the arm stroke and the kick separately and usually very quickly. The most difficult aspect of this skill is learning how to combine these two parts so that maximum performance will result.

When two forces are added sequentially such as in this skill, the exact time that the second force is initiated is most important. If it is started too soon or too late, a decrease in performance will result. Adding this second force at the right time is an example of good coordination.

Coordination has often been referred to as a general motor ability. The reason is that no matter what activity is analyzed, various movements must be integrated if skilled performance

is to be demonstrated. An increase in coordination will result in increased efficiency in the performance of the skill. Coordination is important in all activities.

In activities such as badminton and tennis, hand-eye coordination is very important. A good test to evaluate this component is the alternate-hand wall toss. Three tennis balls, a stop watch, and a smooth-surfaced wall are required for the administration of this test. The subject stands facing the wall, behind a 6-foot restraining line, with a ball held in the right hand. The two extra tennis balls are located in a container at the side of the right foot. At the starting signal the ball is tossed against the wall with an underhand motion and caught in the left hand. It is then thrown with the left hand and caught with the right hand. This movement is repeated as often as possible during a 30-second period. The number of successful catches completed in 30 seconds is counted. The ball must be thrown underhand and cannot be trapped against the body. The restraining line cannot be crossed. One minute of practice is allowed for each subject, followed by two trials.

The results for the alternate-hand wall toss should be recorded:

Trial 1 _____ repetitions
Trial 2 _____ repetitions
Best trial _____ repetitions

Speed and reaction time

Speed is defined as the quickness with which one is able to move his body from one point to another. The distance covered may vary, but in each instance the aim is to move from one point to another in the shortest possible time. Actually, the time taken to perform a task such as this also includes reaction time—defined as the time required to initiate a response to a specific stimulus.[4]

It is generally recognized that speed of movement and the ability to react quickly are of great importance in many different activities. Athletic games and contests abound with illustrations of split-second responses to a stimulus. Keller[5] has shown that when 359 athletes were compared to 277 nonathletes, the athletes were superior to the nonathletes in speed and reaction time. Another study by Tuttle and Westerlund[6] showed also that "outstanding" athletes were superior to "average" athletes in both speed and reaction time.

The sports in which speed and reaction time appear to be most important are baseball, basketball, football, and track. Participants in these sports have been shown to be quicker than participants in gymnastics, wrestling, and swimming.[5] Because of this, students who do not possess above-average speed may have a greater chance of success in the latter three sports than in those of the other group.

Speed can be measured by how fast an individual can move from one point to another. Actually, any distance ranging from 10 to 100-yards can be used for determination of speed. The two distances most frequently used are 50 and 100 yards. Two trials should be given for whichever one of these two tests are used, and the results should be recorded:

_____ yard dash

Trial 1 _____ seconds

Trial 2 _____ seconds

Best trial _____ seconds

Reaction time is defined as the amount of time elapsing between a stimulus and the first movement initiated in response to it. To measure this component, one generally must use special equipment designed for the purpose. However, if a short distance is used for measuring speed, the time will reflect not only the subject's speed but also his reaction time, since both are included in the time taken to complete the performance.

Balance

Balance may be defined as ability to maintain the equilibrium of the body. The two types of balance are static and dynamic. With static balance the equilibrium is maintained in a fixed position, usually while standing on one foot. With dynamic balance the equilibrium must be maintained while performing some task. This might involve walking on a balance beam. The three basic factors that can influence balance are as follows:

1. The height of the center of gravity—the lower the center of gravity, the greater the balance and stability.
2. The size of the base of support—the larger the base of support, the greater the balance and stability.
3. The more nearly centered the line of gravity is to the center of the base of support, the greater the stability.

Balance is important in many different activities and is certainly a contributing factor to skillful performance.

Static balance. This involves any situation in which the body must produce stability and in which no movement takes place. A simple static balance test requires one to assume a diver's stance with the arms outstretched in front, standing on the toes, and with the eyes closed. The aim is to maintain this position as long as possible. This is also one of the items on the 18-item Illinois motor fitness test. To pass this item one must maintain the position for 20 seconds.[2]

Dynamic balance. This involves the maintenance of equilibrium while movement is involved. Many tests are available using the balance beam for evaluation of dynamic balance.

FACTORS THAT INFLUENCE SELECTION OF ACTIVITIES

Many factors influence a person when he decides which activities to participate in. Van Huss et al.[7] list the following:

1. Present emotional needs
2. Present physical needs
3. Present social needs
4. Present interests

5. Future type of work
6. Future place of residence
7. Carry-over values
8. Present level of skills
9. Body type

These factors should be considered by each person, since they can help to make a much wiser decision regarding which activities will be most beneficial now and in the future.

REFERENCES

1. Adams, W. C., Haskell, W. L., Leigh, R. D., Hottinger, W. L., and Penny, W. J.: Foundations of physical activity, Champaign, Ill., Stipes Publishing Co., p. 131.
2. Cureton, T. K.: Run for your life. In The healthy life, New York, 1966, Time, Inc., p. 38.
3. Fleishman, E. A.: The structure and measurement of physical fitness, Englewood Cliffs, N.J., 1964, Prentice-Hall, Inc., p. 29.
4. Johnson, P. B., Updyke, W. F., Stolberg, D. C., and Schaefer, M.: Physical education—a problem solving approach to health and fitness, New York, 1966, Holt, Rinehart and Winston, Inc., p. 26.
5. Keller, L. F.: The relation of quickness of bodily movement to success in athletics, Research Quarterly **13:**146, 1942.
6. Tuttle, W. W., and Westerlund, J. A.: Relationship between running events in track and reaction time, Research Quarterly **2:**95, 1931.
7. Van Huss, W., Niemeyer, R., Olson, H., and Friedrich, J.: Physical activity in modern living, ed. 2, Englewood Cliffs, N.J., 1969, Prentice-Hall, Inc., p. 173.

Name _____ Date _____

Day and hour laboratory section meets _____

Laboratory instructor _____

MOTOR ABILITY PROFILE CHART
Directions

Circle the score closest to the one obtained by you on each test. Connect the circles with a line so that comparisons may be made among the tests.

Men

Percentile rank	AGILITY Agility run (sec)	POWER Standing broad jump (inches)	COORDINATION Alternate-hand wall toss	SPEED 100-yard dash	SPEED 50-yard dash
95	15.0	104	38	11.8	6.1
90	15.6	101	36	12.2	6.2
80	16.3	96	33	12.6	6.4
70	16.8	92	31	12.9	6.5
60	17.2	90	30	13.1	6.6
50	17.6	87	28	13.4	6.8
40	18.0	84	26	13.7	6.9
30	18.4	82	25	13.9	7.0
20	18.9	78	23	14.2	7.1
10	19.6	73	20	14.6	7.5
5	20.2	70	18	15.0	7.7
Mean	17.6	87.0	28.0	13.4	6.8
SD	1.6	10.6	6.3	1.2	.8

Women

Percentile rank	AGILITY Agility run (sec)	POWER Standing broad jump (inches)	COORDINATION Alternate-hand wall toss	SPEED 50-yard dash
95	18.4	77	30	7.3
90	19.1	73	27	7.6
80	19.8	69	24	7.8
70	20.3	66	22	8.0
60	20.8	63	21	8.2
50	21.2	61	19	8.4
40	21.6	59	17	8.7
30	22.1	56	16	9.0
20	22.5	53	14	9.2
10	23.3	49	11	9.7
5	24.0	45	8	10.1
Mean	21.2	61.0	19.0	8.4
SD	1.7	9.5	6.5	.8

Name _____ Date _____

Day and hour laboratory section meets _____

Laboratory instructor _____

SUMMARY SHEET FOR MOTOR ABILITY TEST

Agility run

Trial 1 _____ seconds

Trial 2 _____ seconds

Best trial _____ seconds

Standing broad jump

Trial 1 _____ inches

Trial 2 _____ inches

Best trial _____ inches

Alternate-hand wall toss

Trial 1 _____ repetitions

Trial 2 _____ repetitions

Best trial _____ repetitions

_____-yard dash

Trial 1 _____ seconds

Trial 2 _____ seconds

Best trial _____ seconds

CHAPTER 11

Existing exercise programs

What do you know about existing exercise programs?

T F

☐ ☐   **1.** Any existing exercise program is good and can be used for the optimal development of physical fitness.

☐ ☐   **2.** One of the advantages of the aerobics program is that it is one of the few scientifically developed programs.

☐ ☐   **3.** In the aerobics program most activities are converted to a point system based on the amount of energy expenditure.

☐ ☐   **4.** Tennis is a good activity for the development of cardiovascular endurance.

☐ ☐   **5.** The aim of circuit training is simply to perform a series of calisthenics with rest periods in between.

☐ ☐   **6.** In circuit training each student is competing against each other student.

☐ ☐   **7.** Circuit training does not concentrate on the development of cardiovascular endurance.

☐ ☐   **8.** Progressive overload is built into the circuit training program.

☐ ☐   **9.** Jogging and running are synonymous terms.

☐ ☐   **10.** Low back exercises should aim at the development of the abdominal muscles and stretching of the hamstring muscle group.

☐ ☐   **11.** In the aerobics program the only way a person can earn the required number of points per week is through running, swimming, or riding a bike.

There are many different exercise programs that have been developed and that can be used to develop and maintain an adequate level of physical fitness. Several of these programs will be summarized in this chapter. Students may wish to use these programs in their entirety or adjust the programs to meet their individual needs.

THE AEROBICS PROGRAM

Many times it is of interest to know the individual's capacity for muscular work. This ability to sustain heavy, prolonged muscular work is dependent on the supply of necessary oxygen to the working muscles. *Aerobic work* is thus defined as work performed when sufficient oxygen can be supplied by the body to produce the necessary energy for the performance of the task. Aerobic tasks are those that usually can be maintained for at least 10 minutes and during the performance of which no true oxygen debt is incurred.

The program referred to as *Aerobics* was developed by Dr. Kenneth H. Cooper following 4 years of research using over 15,000 United States Air Force personnel.[2] There really is nothing new concerning the activities that are included in this program, since it utilizes common everyday activities such as walking, running, tennis, and golf. What *is* new about the program is the point system that has been developed as a result of the research. This system allows an individual to equate different activities in terms of energy expenditure and, in this way, to determine *which kinds of activities are best* and also *how long he must participate* in an activity to attain the beneficial results.

This program appears to be designed specifically for the development of the cardiovascular system. A basic assumption underlying this program appears to be that if you develop the cardiovascular system, this will automatically result in the development of "adequate" levels of the other three components of physical fitness—strength, muscular endurance, and flexibility.

In the aerobics program, Cooper was able to equate performance on most activities and then convert this to a point system according to the amount of energy expenditure. The activities that are more strenuous than others were given a higher point value.

Procedures for initiating an aerobics program

Listed are certain procedures that must be followed in order that maximal benefits may be gained from this program:

1. Each participant must know exactly how long he needs to participate in any activity to gain a particular number of points. This is determined by consulting the charts presented by Cooper.
2. Each subject should earn 30 points per week by selecting the work level from any of the available activities. Subjects who have an initially low level of physical fitness should start out by earning only 10 or 15 points per week and increase this work load gradually.
3. A minimum of three or four workouts per week is necessary. To earn all 30 points in one exercise session is not acceptable.
4. An accurate record should be kept of the points earned each day.
5. Periodic evaluation of progress should be made. The 12-minute run test is presented for this purpose, and by periodic use of this a subject can easily measure his progress. This test, of course, can be used to earn points for any day that the subject chooses to use it.

Typical point values for activities

Cooper's findings indicate that the most beneficial activities are running, swimming, cycling, stationary running, handball, and basketball. The amount or rate of work that would need to be performed for several of these activities to achieve certain points is presented in Table 11-1.

His findings also indicated that activities such

Table 11-1. Point values for certain selected activities in the aerobics program

Running (time for 1 mile)	Running (time for 2 miles)	Handball or basketball*	Swimming (time for 400 yards)	Cycling (time for 3 miles)	Points
More than 20 min	—	Less than 8 min	—	18 min or longer	0
14½-20 min	40 min or longer	8 min	13½ min or longer	12-17 min	1
12-14½ min	29-40 min	15 min	10-13½ min	—	2
10-12 min	—	20 min	7-9 min	9-11 min	3
8-10 min	24-28 min	28 min	—	—	4
6½-8 min	—	35 min	Less than 7 min	Less than 9 min	5
Less than 6½ min	20-24 min	40 min	—	—	6

*The times for handball and basketball are for continuous activity and do not include breaks, etc.; must also be full court basketball.

Table 11-2. Point values for certain additional exercises in the aerobics program

Activity	Amount of activity	Points
Golf (no motorized carts)	18 holes	3
Hockey*	20 min	3
Rope skipping (continuous)	5 min	1½
Skating*	15 min	1
Skiing*	30 min	3
Tennis	1 set	1½
Volleyball*	15 min	1
Wrestling*	5 min	2

*Only the time that is spent actively is to be counted.

as weight lifting, calisthenics, and isometrics did not contribute to the development of cardiovascular endurance, whereas sports such as golf, tennis, and volleyball produced very *minimal* contributions. The point values assigned to performance in several of these activities are presented in Table 11-2.

Laboratory experience

In the laboratory session or sessions devoted to explaining this program, each student should experience a number of different ways of earning an approximately equal number of points. In this way, the relative strenuousness of the activities can be compared by each individual. Also each person is introduced to different activities that can be used as part of this program. The instructor and the students may wish to select any number of the activities suggested in Table 11-3. The facilities available may dictate the activities that can be covered during the laboratory period. This work will be more meaningful if three or four different activities are used during the session. For additional activities, the reader is referred to the tables contained in *The New Aerobics*.

Most individuals find participating in activities such as tennis, golf, badminton, skiing, and skating more enjoyable than running, jumping rope continuously, or running in place for extended periods of time. If this is the case, it seems important for an individual to develop a skill level in at least one physical activity that could be used later in life, particularly when the student leaves college. Ideally, this activity should involve only one or two persons, and the more vigorous the activity is, the more beneficial it will be. Also, the skill level that is devel-

Table 11-3. Suggested activities to be used for comparative purposes

Activity	Duration	Points
Rope skipping (continuous)	5 min	1½
Volleyball	23 min	1½
Basketball	10 min	1½
Stationary running	5 min (must complete approximately 350 steps*)	1½
Running/walking	1 mile in 12 min	2

*Count only when the left foot hits the floor.

oped is a very important consideration. One's own skill level and that of the opponent determines to a large extent the vigorousness of the activity and the rate of energy expenditure.

CIRCUIT TRAINING

Circuit training is a form of general fitness training that evolved out of a search for a method that would both appeal to the students and also measurably increase their physical fitness level. It is based on sound physiological principles and was developed at the University of Leeds in 1955.[8]

The term *circuit* refers to a given number of exercises arranged and numbered consecutively in a given area. Each numbered exercise within the circuit is referred to as a *station*. The type of circuit that is set up is dependent on the time, space, and facilities available and the objectives desired for the program. The stations are usually located at approximately equal distances from each other and are designated by signs on the walls or bleachers that might surround the given area where the circuit is set up. These signs indicate the sequence for the activities and also the prescribed number of repetitions at each station.

The activities included in the circuit can be selected to achieve almost any objective in an attempt to develop the physical fitness components or the motor ability components or a combination of both. Also a circuit that is directed entirely to the development of specific skills can be set up.

Objectives

In circuit training each subject progresses at his own rate from one station to the next, performing a prescribed amount of work at each, until the entire circuit has been completed. Usually the single circuit is repeated several times, and the time for the total performance is recorded. The participants proceed from station to station without resting as they attempt to reduce the time taken for a given number of laps around the circuit. The basic assumption underlying circuit training is that improvement takes place either by doing the same amount of work in a shorter period of time or by doing more work in a given period of time. A student can progress by decreasing the time required to complete a given number of laps of the circuit or by increasing the number of repetitions performed at each station or by a combination of both of these methods.

The principle of progressive overload is stressed with circuit training. This principle is explained simply by Steinhaus:

No matter how much a muscle is used, it will not grow larger or stronger until it is overloaded. This means that the intensity of the work required of it must be increased above that to which it is currently accustomed, i.e. it must be required to exert more power or work against a greater resistance than before.[12]

With circuit training, a progressive overload is built into the program by increasing the amount of work, increasing the rate of work, or decreasing the time factor.

Advantages

The basic advantage over other methods or calisthenics or programs of exercise is that circuit training stresses *continuous activity*. It has already been shown that continuous activity is a prerequisite for the development of the cardiovascular system. Unfortunately many of the exercise programs available today stress only muscular endurance and flexibility and place little emphasis on the development of cardiovascular endurance. Sorani[11] indicates that many students perform exercises of one type or another and that these exercises, if performed regularly and properly, can be worthwhile and satisfying. However, he indicates that frequently exercise programs are not well planned or organized and that little thought is given to their purpose or procedure. Also many students participate in these exercise programs only when they like. When exercise is not performed on a regular basis, it is very difficult to include progressive overloading because lack of activity on a regular basis may result in regression. With circuit training, however, progression is built into the program, and each student should be working at his present capacity, since he progresses at his own rate. Circuit training, however, is no different from any other form of training in that the results depend entirely on the effort put forth by each participant.

Following is a list of the advantages associated with circuit training:

1. Each participant is able to commence this program at an easy pace and to experience some degree of success early in the program.
2. Circuit training can be organized so as to involve a large number of students in a relatively confined area.
3. Added motivation is provided by the fact that each participant can see his progress from day to day.
4. Progression is assured if the participant exercises regularly.
5. With circuit training the exercise is continuous, and thus stress is placed on the cardiovascular system.
6. Circuit training provides for individualized self-competition. Each participant is competing only against himself, and he works at his own individual rate.

Organization

Circuit training may be organized in a variety of different ways. Following is an example of the organization of a circuit consisting of 11 stations designed to develop the overall physical fitness of freshmen at the university level. This circuit is applicable for men and women students. A list of the activities and the repeti-

Table 11-4. Circuit training activities

	I Yellow	II Black	III Red	IV Blue
1. Lateral jump	25	30	35	50
2. Hip raiser	10	12	16	25
3. Bent-leg sit-ups	10	15	20	30
4. Rope jump	40	50	60	80
5. Lateral leg raise	8	10	20	30
6. Burpee	8	10	20	30
7. Alternate toe-touch	20	25	35	40
8. V-sits	10	14	18	24
9. Push-ups	8	12	20	30
10. Bench jump	10	16	20	26
11. Sprinter	20	30	40	50

tions for each of these are presented in Table 11-4.

Four progression levels have been established, although more may be added if they are needed. The initial starting level for each person can be determined by his performance on the 12-minute run test. Table 11-5 presents the criteria to be used in the determination of the starting level for each student. If the student has not taken this test, starting him at the lowest level and letting him progress from there is probably best.

Description of activities included in the circuit*

Lateral jump. Each subject jumps laterally across any line on the floor as fast as possible,

*Several of these exercises are adapted from or similar to those suggested by Robert Sorani in his book *Circuit Training*, Dubuque, Iowa, 1966, Wm. C. Brown Co., pp. 45-62.

keeping both feet together and parallel to the line. This activity develops muscular endurance of the legs as well as overall cardiovascular endurance.

Hip raiser. Each subject assumes the starting position as shown in Fig. 11-1. The hips are elevated as high as possible and then lowered as low as possible without the buttocks touching the floor. This exercise will develop the muscular endurance of certain hip and thigh muscles as well as the abdominal muscles. It can be a good exercise to correct drooping shoulders.

Bent-leg sit-ups. This exercise is designed to strengthen the abdominal muscles and to increase their endurance. Each subject lies on his back on the floor with knees flexed at approximately 90° and feet placed flat on the floor. Flexing the knees places more stress on the abdominal muscles, and the muscles that flex the hip contribute less to the exercise. The fingers

Table 11-5. Criteria for determination of the initial starting level for circuit training

Classification for 12-minute run test	Distance covered (miles)		Initial circuit level
	Men	Women	
Very poor or poor	Less than 1.24	Less than 1.19	Level I—Yellow circuit
Average	1.25-1.53	1.20-1.27	Level II—Black circuit
Good	1.57-1.84	1.28-1.42	Level III—Red circuit
Excellent	More than 1.84	More than 1.43	Level IV—Blue circuit

Fig. 11-1. Starting position for the hip raiser exercise.

are interlocked and placed behind the neck (Fig. 6-1). The subject sits up so that at least one elbow touches one knee each time and then returns to the starting position. Each time he returns to the starting position, the fingers at the back of the head must come in contact with the floor.

Rope jump. This activity is designed for the development of cardiovascular endurance. A regular jump rope is used, and each subject must propel the rope in a counterclockwise direction so that it passes under his feet and over his head. Each time the rope passes under the feet counts as one repetition.

Lateral leg raise. Each subject assumes a position on the floor lying on either side with legs and lower arm completely extended and using the other arm to maintain his balance (Fig. 11-2). The upper leg is raised as high as possible, being kept straight, and is then returned slowly to the starting position. This constitutes one repetition. This exercise is designed to develop the muscles responsible for abduction of the leg. If the circuit is completed more than one time, the sides should be reversed, so that the leg that is raised is changed each time around the circuit.

Burpee. This exercise is also referred to as the squat-thrust or the agility 4-count exercise. Each subject starts in a standing position with the legs straight. He assumes the squat position, extends the legs backward so that he assumes the push-up position, then reverses this procedure back to the squat position and finally back to the upright position. This completes one repetition. Because this exercise involves many large muscle groups, it contributes to overall muscular endurance.

Alternate toe-touch. This exercise is a flexibility exercise designed to increase trunk flexion. Again the subject assumes an upright standing position with legs straight and feet shoulder-width apart. The arms are extended above the head. Keeping the legs straight, he reaches down to touch the left foot with the right hand, then returns to the starting position before reaching down again to touch the right foot with the left hand. When he returns again to the starting position, he has completed one repetition.

V-sits. The subject lies on the floor on his back at the start of this activity with arms extended fully behind the head. He then curls the head toward the chest as the arms and legs are

Fig. 11-2. Lateral leg exercise.

Fig. 11-3. V-sit position.

raised simultaneously until a V-position is attained (Fig. 11-3). The subject then reverses these procedures until the starting position is reached. This exercise is a good one for the development of the abdominal muscles, particularly if the V-position is maintained for a few seconds each time.

Push-ups. Men should perform the regular push-up, starting from the front-leaning rest position with the head, back, hips, and legs in a straight alignment. The body is slowly lowered so that the chest lightly touches the floor. The body should remain straight throughout this exercise. The arms are then extended as the body is raised to the starting position. This exercise will develop the muscular endurance and strength of the extensors of the forearm. Women should perform the modified push-up (Fig. 11-4) or the alternate method for the push-up, using the lowest row of bleachers for support (Fig. 11-5).

Bench jump or bench step. For this activity the subject faces a bench that is approximately 12 to 16 inches high. The lowest row of bleach-

ers is usually satisfactory for this exercise. The subject jumps up onto and down from the bench. This completes one repetition. If he is unable to jump onto the bench, he should step up, following the same procedure that is used for the step test. This exercise is designed to develop cardiovascular endurance as well as strength and endurance of the leg extensors.

Sprinter. The subject assumes a position similar to a sprinter's starting position, with the weight on the hands and feet with one leg extended straight back and the other flexed with the knee pulled under the chest (Fig. 11-6). The position of the feet is then reversed and reversed again as the subject returns to the starting position. This completes one repetition. This exercise contributes to the development of strength and endurance of the shoulder and arm extensors as well as leg flexors and extensors.

Instructions for running a circuit

All students should be provided with the following information before the circuit is attempted. In addition, each exercise should be

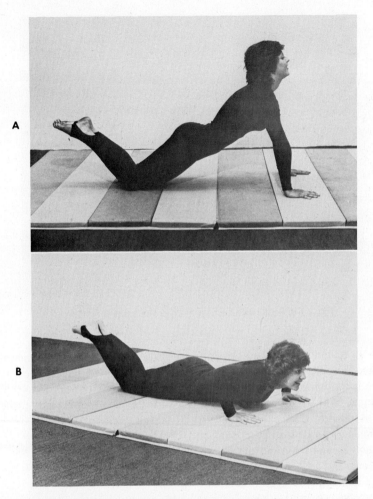

Fig. 11-4. Starting **(A)** and finishing **(B)** positions for the modified push-up for women.

Fig. 11-5. Alternate method of push-ups for women.

Fig. 11-6. Position to be assumed for the sprinter exercise.

demonstrated to the students, and they should each have a chance to practice the exercise so that it may be performed correctly.

1. Fifteen minutes will be allowed for each male and 18 minutes for each female student to complete two laps of the circuit.
2. If the two laps around the circuit are completed before the allocated time has elapsed, the remainder of the time is to be spent completing as many single laps across the badminton court as are possible in the remaining time. The same procedures that apply to the 3-minute shuttle run will apply here. These procedures are outlined in Chapter 5.
3. If a subject completes 20 or more laps within the time limit, the next time he attempts the circuit, he should move up to the next level.
4. A person who fails to complete two entire laps of the circuit in the prescribed time and is not working at level I should move back one level the next time that he attempts the circuit.
5. To measure progress each day each stu-

dent should record the total time taken to complete two laps of the circuit and also the number of laps across the badminton court completed within the prescribed time limit.

WALKING-JOGGING-RUNNING PROGRAM

Running as a method for the development of physical fitness is looked upon unfavorably by many people. However "such an image of running only reflects a poor understanding of this versatile means of activity. Running as a means of obtaining a feeling of well-being need not, and should not, be an unpleasant experience nor should it be a daily challenge of man's ability to survive physical adversity."*

Definition of terms

Certain terms must be defined for a clear understanding of the following material that is presented in this unit:

*From Balke, B.: Guidelines for walking-jogging-running training mimeographed material, Madison, University of Wisconsin, p. 1. Portions of this discussion are summarized from this material.

Walking—form of movement in which at least one foot is in contact with the ground at all times

Jogging—form of running, at a slow to moderate pace; Balke clarifies this definition by stating that "jogging is running at a speed which can be equalled or surpassed by fast walking"

Running—form of movement during which no more than one foot may be in contact with the ground at any one time or both feet are off the ground during a portion of each stride

Interval running—intermittent running in which a given distance is repeated several times with a rest interval between each run; the "rest" may be in the form of walking, jogging, or complete rest

Brisk walking, jogging, or running may be used for a variety of reasons. Probably the fundamental purpose is to increase one's cardiovascular endurance. By progressively making the task more difficult, the development of the circulatory system takes place, and the body is capable of using more oxygen.[4]

Secondary objectives as presented by Roby and Davis[9] include "the improvement of appearance through weight or figure control and better posture, together with improvement of those psychological traits which have to do with inner confidence, will-power and the ability to resist both mental and physical stress."

Variation of the program

The strenuousness of the program can be varied by any one of the following: (1) regulating the distance covered, (2) adjusting the ratio of walking to running, or (3) adjusting the speed of running. The program needs to be adapted to the age and fitness levels of the participants as realistic objectives are established.

Advantages of a jogging program*

Following is a list of advantages associated with a well-designed jogging or running program:

1. Simple and most effective way to stimu-

---

*The material in this section is summarized from *Running Into Fitness*, a pamphlet produced by the National Fitness Council of South Australia.

late the circulation and exercise the heart.

2. Superior to many other forms of exercise in that it provides a gentle, steady, and prolonged demand on the heart rather than a series of short but severe ones.
3. Provides for the development of body flexibility and exercises most parts of the body.
4. Can be adapted to the physical fitness and age level of each participant.
5. Can be performed at any time and place.
6. Requires no special equipment or facilities, and the costs involved are very minimal.
7. Takes little time.
8. Requires little learning skill, since it is a natural activity.

Development of a jogging program

In designing a jogging or running program the following guidelines may be helpful:[10]

1. Begin by walking daily, increasing the speed of walking until you can walk briskly for 10 minutes without overexertion.
2. Next, alternate jogging with walking for a total of 10 minutes daily. Gradually increase the amount of jogging as you spend less time walking until you are able to jog continuously for 10 minutes.
3. Finally, increase the length of time spent jogging daily and also increase the speed of jogging as your endurance increases. You will progress from jogging to running.
4. You need to run at least every second day. If you can make this 5 or 6 days per week, the training effects should occur much more quickly.
5. It is not important to concentrate on running style, but beginners should try placing the ball and heel of the foot first and not the toes. Relaxation of the ankles, knees, hips, shoulders, face, and hands should also be considered. The more relaxed the person is, the easier it is for him to run.

For further details concerning standardized jogging and running programs that have been developed for persons of all ages, see the program suggested by Bowerman and Harris[1] or the program by Roby and Davis.[9]

Changes that take place as a result of jogging and running

A report by Wilmore[13] indicates that jogging is an excellent form of exercise, provided that a medical examination is obtained before the beginning of the program, the program is started gradually, and each participant avoids competing with his friends. He indicated that as a result of an 11-week jogging program, the following changes resulted: (1) an 8% decrease in body fat, (2) a significant increase in vital capacity, (3) a 10% to 13% decrease in resting blood pressure, (4) a 12% decrease in the resting heart rate, and (5) a significant decrease in the cholesterol and triglyceride levels.

INTERVAL TRAINING

Not all exercise programs need to be performed continuously. For example, in an exercise program designed to lose weight, the total amount of work performed is most important. The more work that is performed, the more Calories are used, and thus the greater the loss in weight. Whether this work is performed continuously is not important. It has been shown clearly that when a task is broken up into bouts of short duration with intervening periods of rest, greater total work loads can be performed. This type of training is referred to as interval training.[2] Actually, there are four variables involved with interval training, any one or all of which can be altered to change the intensity of the task—(1) the distance to be run, (2) the amount of time taken to run this distance, (3) the number of times this distance is to be run (repetitions), and (4) the amount of time allowed for rest between each run. An example should help to make this information more meaningful. Interval training for a specific situation might involve running four repetitions of 100 yards each, at full speed, with a 20-second rest interval between each bout. Any one or all of the four variables could be altered to change the intensity of the task. A much more strenuous task might be running eight repetitions of 220 yards each in 45 seconds with a 2-minute rest interval between each repetition. With this task, if a participant takes less than 45 seconds to run the 220 yards, he has the additional time added to his rest period. A person who takes longer than 45 seconds to run the 220 yards would actually have less than a 2-minute rest between repetitions.

Laboratory experience

The laboratory work that each person can experience with this unit will vary according to the facilities available. Following are several suggestions that might be included:

1. Each student should jog continuously at a comfortable pace for a 10-minute period. The pace will be determined by each student, and at the completion of the jog he should feel comfortable and not be exhausted. Each subject should calculate the distance covered, and the point table (Table 12-1) should be consulted to determine how many points this would earn in the aerobics program. It should be stressed that the aim of this is *not* to cover the greatest possible distance but merely to establish a comfortable jogging speed for a 10-minute period of time.

Distance covered in 10 minutes
at a moderate jogging speed = _____ miles
Speed = _____ miles
× 6
Speed = _____miles/hr

2. Each student can be introduced to an interval training program designed to develop speed and power. Each student should select at least one of the following tasks[6]:

a. Ten repetitions of 100 yards each in 18

seconds with 110-yard walk interval between each run
b. Twenty repetitions of 60 yards each in 9
seconds with a 30-second rest interval between each run
c. Thirty repetitions of 40 yards each in 6
seconds with a 20-second rest interval between each run

3. Each student can participate in an interval-
training program designed to develop cardiovascular endurance. Again each instructor or
class should select at least one of the following
tasks[4]:
a. Three repetitions of 880 yards each in 3½
minutes with a 5-minute rest interval between each run
b. Six repetitions of 440 yards each in 100
seconds with a 2-minute rest interval between each run
c. Two repetitions of 1 mile each in 9 minutes with a 3-minute rest interval between
each run

Summary

There are many different methods available
to vary the walking-jogging-running program.
By varying the program from day to day, each
person is much more likely to maintain his initial motivation. Remember that walking, jogging, and running can be a lot of fun.

EXERCISE PROGRAM FOR ALLEVIATION OF LOW BACK PAIN

It has been clearly demonstrated that the
great majority of persons who suffer from low
back pain can alleviate the problem by regular
exercise. However, the choice of exercises is
very important. Ones that will strengthen the
abdominal musculature and lengthen the hamstring muscle group must be selected. Kraus[6]
has shown that the following exercises are most
beneficial in the elimination of low back pain:

1. *Bent-knee sit-ups*. Instructions are the same as
those for item 2 of the Kraus-Weber test.
2. *Toe touches*. The instructions for this activity are
the same as those for item 6 of the Kraus-Weber
test.
3. *Back hyperextension*. The subject assumes a
prone position with a pillow under his pelvis.
With feet held and arms straight and at his side,
the upper body is lifted off the floor until the legs
and body are in a straight line.
4. *Back arch*. The subject assumes a kneeling position on "all fours" on the floor. The back is
arched upward as far as possible from the floor. In
this position the head should be lowered so that
the forehead is as close to the floor as possible.
Next, the back is "dropped" to a swayback position, and the head is lifted so that the forehead is
as far away from the floor as possible.
5. *Leg curls*. The subject assumes a supine position
on the floor. With hands behind the neck, the legs
are slowly lifted, the knees are bent, and the legs
are curled until the knees are in contact with the
chest. The legs are then straightened and lowered
to the starting position.

Other exercise programs are available for al-
leviation of low back pain and for building a
stronger back. Feffer suggests that the following eight exercises be performed twice a day,
starting with four repetitions and increasing to
ten. The exercises he recommends are as follows:

Lying on stomach
1. Pinch buttocks together. Pull stomach in. Hold
position for 5 seconds, then relax 5 seconds.
Over a period of days, increase holding-relax-
ing period to 20 seconds.

Lying on back
2. Bend knees with feet flat on floor, keeping
arms at sides. Pinch buttocks together. Pull in
stomach and flatten lower back against floor.
Hold for 5 seconds, relax for 5 seconds. Gradually build up to 20 seconds.
3. Repeat exercise 2 with legs extended.
4. Draw knees toward chest. Clasp hands around
knees. Keep shoulders flat against floor. Pull
knees tightly against chest, then bring forehead
to knees.
5. Bend knees with feet flat on floor; cross arms
on chest. Raise head and shoulders from floor.
Curl up to sitting position. Keep back round

and pull with stomach muscles. Lower self slowly.

6. Bend knees, keep feet flat on floor and arms straight forward. Touch head to knees. Lower self. Draw knees toward chest. Pull knees tightly against chest and bring forehead to knees.

Sitting on floor

7. Keep legs straight. Pull stomach in. Reach forward with hands and try to touch toes with fingers. Use rocking motion.

Sitting on a chair

8. Place hands at edge of chair. Bend forward to bring head to knees, pulling stomach in as you curl forward. Keep weight well back on hips. Release stomach muscles slowly as you come up.*

---

*Reprinted from U.S. News & World Report, Sept. 20, 1971. Copyright 1971 U.S. News & World Report, Inc.

REFERENCES

1. Bowerman, W. J., and Harris, W. E.: Jogging, New York, 1967, Grosset & Dunlap, Inc.
2. Cooper, K. H.: New aerobics, New York, 1972, Bantam Books, Inc.
3. DeVries, H. A.: Physiology of exercise for physical education and athletics, ed. 4, London, 1968, Staples Press, Ltd., pp. 219, 333-335.
4. Harris, W. E., and Bowerman, W.: Jogging—an adult exercise program, The Journal of the American Medical Association **201:**759, 1967.
5. Howell, M. L., and Morford, W. R.: Circuit training for a college fitness program, Journal of Health, Physical Education and Recreation **35:**30, 1964.
6. Kraus, H.: Backache, stress, and tension; their cause, prevention, and treatment, New York, 1965, Simon & Schuster, Inc.
7. Landers, D., and Wade, M.: The University of Illinois foundations laboratory handbook.
8. Morgan, R. E., and Adamson, G. T.: Circuit training, London, 1957, G. Bell & Sons, Ltd.
9. Roby, F. B., and Davis, R. P.: Jogging for fitness and weight control, Philadelphia, 1970, W. B. Saunders Company, pp. 1-109.
10. Run for your life program provokes a physician debate, Medical Tribune, Oct. 12, 1967.
11. Sorani, R.: Circuit training, Dubuque, Iowa, 1966, Wm. C. Brown Company, Publishers, pp. 45-62.
12. Steinhaus, A. H.: Strength from Mofungo to Mueller—a half century of research, Journal of the Association for Physical and Mental Rehabilitation **9:**147, Sept.-Oct., 1955.
13. Wilmore, J. H.: Benefits derived from an 11-week jogging program, Medicine in Sports, p. 4, Nov. 9, 1969.

CHAPTER 12

Relative value of various activities in the development of physical fitness

What do you know about the contribution of various activities to the development of physical fitness?

T F

☐ ☐ **1.** For an activity to contribute to the development of physical fitness it must produce a near-maximal heart rate.

☐ ☐ **2.** Maximal heart rate will not change drastically as one ages.

☐ ☐ **3.** Activities that require continuous action and involve large muscle groups will generally be good for the development of cardiovascular endurance.

☐ ☐ **4.** Tennis is a good activity for the development of cardiovascular endurance.

☐ ☐ **5.** One of the best activities for the development of cardiovascular endurance is basketball.

☐ ☐ **6.** An activity must produce a heart rate of 140 to 150 beats per minute and sustain this for 5 minutes to be beneficial for the development of cardiovascular endurance.

☐ ☐ **7.** Football is a very poor activity for the development of cardiovascular fitness.

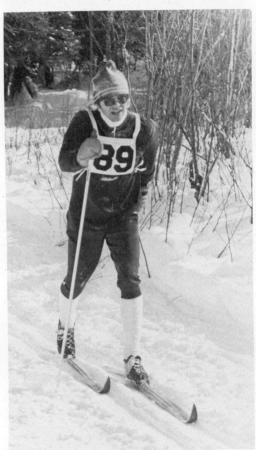

In designing an exercise program, it is important to know how strenuous an activity must be to contribute toward the development of cardiovascular fitness and which activities can best be used for this purpose.

CRITICAL HEART RATE

It has been shown that if an activity is to contribute to the development of cardiovascular fitness, there is a critical heart rate that must be exceeded. Working with untrained subjects, Karvonen[5] found that if an activity is to improve the exercise tolerance of the heart, it must produce a heart rate in excess of the value located 60% of the way between the resting and the maximal heart rates. For most of these subjects, this critical value was between 140 and 150 beats per minute. The resting heart rate may be determined very easily. This should be taken several times to make sure that the value

is a typical value for the subject involved. The maximal heart rate can be estimated as follows:

Estimated maximal heart rate = 220 − age (years)

= 220 − _____

= _____

Resting heart rate = _____ Trial 1

= _____ Trial 2

= _____ Trial 3

= _____ Trial 4

Typical score = _____ beats/ minute

Evaluation of critical heart rate

Critical heart rate = Resting heart rate + .60 (Maximal heart rate − Resting heart rate)

EXAMPLE: If a subject has a resting heart rate of 70 beats per minute and a maximal heart rate of 190 beats per minute . . .

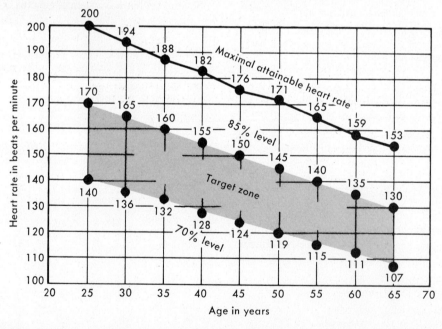

Fig. 12-1. Summary of changes that take place as a result of age as far as the maximal attainable heart rate is concerned and what the target zone is for each age group. The numerical values shown are "average" values for each age. (Courtesy Best Foods Division, CPC International, Englewood Cliffs, N.J.)

Critical heart rate = 70 + .60 (190 − 70)

= 70 + .60 (120)

= 70 + 72

= 142

Each person should calculate his own critical heart rate.

Critical heart rate = _____ + .60 (_____ − _____)

= _____ + .60 (_____)

= _____ + _____

= _____

Cooper[2] has indicated that for maximal development of cardiovascular endurance an activity must produce a heart rate in excess of 150 beats per minute and that improvement begins only after this rate of activity has been sustained for at least 5 minutes. In addition to this, the activity must be performed a minimum of three or four times per week.

The American Heart Association[8] suggests that there is a target zone as far as heart rate is concerned that is sufficient to develop cardiovascular fitness but not too high to exceed safe limits. This suggested target zone is between 70% and 85% of a person's maximal aerobic power. Below 70% of his capacity, a person achieves very little fitness benefit, while above 85% there is very little added benefit. The maximal attainable heart rates and the target zones for different age groups are presented in Fig. 12-1.

RELATIVE STRENUOUSNESS OF VARIOUS ACTIVITIES

To learn which activities are most stressful to the heart and can be used for the development of cardiovascular endurance is important. Identifying activities that are less stressful also is important. This information allows the individual to increase the efficiency of his heart by overloading it at times and allowing it to slow down at other times.

In activities such as running, swimming, and bicycling the strenuousness will be determined by how fast one performs. This, of course, is related to how much time is taken to cover a specified distance. The reader is referred to tables in the Cooper book that have been based on these criteria.

DETERMINATION OF THE STRENUOUSNESS OF AN ACTIVITY

Without some form of telemetry equipment, it is difficult to determine the heart rate during participation in most activities. An alternate method is to determine the pulse immediately upon completing the exercise. It is important to count immediately because the rate changes very quickly once exercise is slowed or stopped. The American Heart Association recommends that you find the beat within 1 second of the end of exercise, count for 10 seconds, and multiply this by 6 to convert this to beats per minute. They suggest that this is superior to counting for the whole minute or for 15 seconds because the "drop-off" is too fast.

Several studies have been conducted comparing different activities. Balke[1] has conducted research comparing 11 different activities. In this study the maximum capacity is expressed in Mets. One Met is equivalent to the energy a person uses while sitting at rest. The 11 activities are listed in Table 12-1 in order of the maximal capacity in Mets.

Table 12-1. Maximal capacity in Mets of athletes[3]

Sport	Maximal capacity in Mets
Track running	23
Cross country skiing	23
Speed skating	23
Rowing	19
Cycling	18
Competitive swimming	18
Alpine skiing	16
Ice hockey	16
Basketball	15½
Tennis	13
Football	13

The National Athletic Health Institute[6] has released figures comparing various groups of male athletes. Their unit for comparative purposes is maximal oxygen uptake expressed in milliliters of oxygen per kilogram of body weight (ml/kg Bw). The maximal oxygen uptake of an individual represents the best estimate available for cardiovascular fitness and endurance capacity. The reason for this is that all living cells require oxygen to function properly, and as muscular activity is increased, the oxygen demanded by the muscles increases in direct proportion. There is a definite limit with regard to how much oxygen your body can supply. Theoretically, the higher this value, the higher the level of cardiovascular fitness.

Maximal oxygen uptake figures for 12 different sports are provided in Table 12-2.

The results presented in Table 12-2 show that the five sports that rank highest all require continuous sustained action over a long period of time and involve the use of large muscle groups.

The sports that ranked near the bottom of the list, such as football, baseball and tennis, do not involve continuous activity. In tennis it was found that more than 50% of the time was spent standing around getting ready to play and *not* in actual competition.

A similar comparison was conducted by Golding[7] at Kent State University. He compared 10 different sports and ranked them according to the level of cardiovascular fitness of participants. His rankings were as follows: (1) track, (2) swimming, (3) cross-country, (4) soccer, (5) ice hockey, (6) basketball, (7) football, (8) tennis, (9) baseball, and (10) golf.

Several studies have shown that neither golf nor weight lifting produces a heart rate in excess of the threshold value required to produce a training effect. Weight lifters, despite their well-developed skeletal system, rate no higher in cardiovascular endurance than the average untrained subject. Getchell[4] studied the effect of a season of golf for 20 middle-aged golfers who averaged more than 12 hours per week on the golf course. When compared to the sedentary group of subjects, there was very little difference in their response to a submaximal work task.

Activities can be classified into four groups according to the contributions they might make toward the development of cardiovascular fitness. These arbitary classifications are as follows:

Table 12-2. Maximal oxygen uptake in milliliters per kilogram of body weight in males

Sport	Maximal O$_2$ uptake (average figures— ml O$_2$/kg Bw)
Cross country skiing	70-94
Long distance running	65-85
Rowing	58-75
Bicycling	55-70
Basketball	55-70
Speed skating	50-75
Ice hockey	50-60
Distance swimming	48-68
Gymnastics	48-64
Football	45-64
Baseball	45-55
Tennis	42-56

Group 1:
Low contribution
Archery
Bowling
Baseball
Calisthenics
Golf
Volleyball

Group 2:
Minimal contribution
Gymnastics
Tennis
Football

Group 3:
High contribution
Badminton
Basketball
Rowing
Judo
Snowshoeing

Group 4:
Very high contribution
Bicycling
Handball
Paddleball
Squash
Running
Soccer
Swimming
Cross-country skiing
Wrestling

SUMMARY

Various studies clearly indicate that activities involving continuous activity and large muscle groups can be used to develop cardiovascular endurance. Activities that result in a heart rate in excess of 140 to 150 beats per minute and that are continued for extended periods of time appear to be most beneficial. Research indicates that activities such as running, cross-country skiing, skating, rowing, bicycling, swimming, hiking, handball, paddleball, basketball, and orienteering are some of the activities that rate high. Activities such as weight lifting, football, volleyball, golf, and calisthenics rate low when evaluated according to these criteria.

REFERENCES

1. Balke, B.: Rank of apparent benefits of various activities in Mets. Proceedings of American College of Sports Medicine, May, 1971.
2. Cooper, K.: Aerobics, New York, 1968, M. Evans and Company, Inc.
3. Cundiff, D. E.: Fundamentals of functional fitness, Dubuque, Iowa, 1974, Kendall/Hunt Publishing Company, p. 67.
4. Getchell, L. H., Energy cost of playing golf, Archives of Physical Medicine **49:**31-35, Jan. 1968.
5. Karvonen, M. J.: Effects of vigorous exercise on the heart. In Rosenbaum, F. F., and Belknap, E. L., editors: Work and the heart, New York, 1959, Paul B. Hoeber, Inc.
6. National Athletic Health Institute, printed information, California, 1975.
7. Newsletter: President's Council on Physical Fitness and Sports, Washington, D.C., Aug.-Sept., 1973, p. 4.
8. Zohman, L. R.: Exercise your way to fitness and heart health, American Heart Association, 1974, p. 11.

CHAPTER 13

Developing an exercise program

What do you know about developing an exercise program?

T F

☐ ☐ **1.** Exercising for 1 hour per week is as beneficial as exercising for 10 minutes daily.

☐ ☐ **2.** Progressive resistance is no longer necessary once a desired level of fitness has been reached.

☐ ☐ **3.** Overload is a form of physical stress.

☐ ☐ **4.** Intensity and duration of physical exercises provide the primary means by which activity may become progressively more strenuous.

T F

☐ ☐ **5.** An overload is any exercise that exceeds in intensity or duration the demands usually made on the organism.

☐ ☐ **6.** Most existing exercise programs are good for the development of cardiovascular fitness.

☐ ☐ **7.** A person must exercise every day if he wants to improve his level of physical fitness.

☐ ☐ **8.** A person need only exercise 10 minutes per day to bring about maximal development of physical fitness.

The preceding chapters have presented information relative to the importance of regular physical activity. The reasons for maintaining a desirable level of physical fitness and body weight have been discussed. Along with this information, a series of tests was also presented so that each individual could carefully evaluate his present level of fitness, motor ability, and nutritional status. Several different exercise programs have been summarized that can be used for improving one's level of fitness.

All this information has been presented in the hope that persons may realize just how unfit they really are and may do something about it. Having knowledge about physical fitness is not sufficient; the knowledge must be applied and used. Each person must believe strongly enough in the importance of physical fitness to do something about it. Knowing and talking about it are not sufficient.

PRINCIPLES OF EXERCISE

There are certain basic principles that need to be followed if a good exercise program is to result.

1. *It takes time and effort to develop an adequate level of physical fitness.* No "short-cut," easy methods exist. Cureton states that "the first thing you must do is to face the fact that there are no short cuts. It will take three months of hard work—possibly the hardest work of your life—before you see significant changes."[1] For this reason the development of physical fitness should be a lifetime matter. Ideally, an adequate level of physical fitness should be developed early and be maintained throughout life.[3] It has been suggested that physical fitness should be considered as a continuum or scale (Fig. 3-2). The amount and type of physical activity that each person includes in his daily routine will determine to a large extent his position on this scale. If exercise is not continued throughout life, there will be a decrease in the level of physical fitness.

2. *The program should be designed to meet the present needs of the individual.* Much time and energy can be wasted unless certain specific goals are established for a program. These goals should be based on the needs of each individual. It has been emphasized that the level of physical fitness necessary will vary. Some persons need a much higher level of physical fitness than others.

After an individual has established his specific goals, he must be able to evaluate carefully his progress as he strives to attain his objectives. There is no exercise program that is good for everyone. Each has to be designed to suit the needs, abilities, and goals of each person.

3. *A well-planned program will be directed toward the improvement of each component of physical fitness.* It has been emphasized that physical fitness involves strength, flexibility, and muscular and cardiovascular endurance. A good exercise program must be directed toward the development of all four components. It has also been stressed that of these four components cardiovascular endurance is the most important health benefit. Therefore the development of this component should occupy a prominent position in any exercise program.

4. *The program must be systematic.* All too frequently exercise is performed irregularly, with little thought given to the reasons for specific exercises. Exercises must be organized into a systematic program designed to meet the basic needs of each individual.

5. *Regular participation in any exercise program is necessary.* To achieve specific objectives, participation must be on a regular basis. Persons who wait until they "find" time to exercise do not exercise very often. If they believe strongly enough in the importance of exercise, they will make time available on a regular basis. Exercise should become a habit, and if possible, it should be scheduled at a regular time each day. An exercise program can be considered regular when participation occurs at least four times a week.

6. *An overload is the key to a successful*

program. For significant improvement to take place, an overload is necessary—meaning simply that it is necessary to subject the body to a task slightly beyond its normal level. DeVries indicates that "whether we are concerned with strength, muscular endurance, or cardiovascular endurance, improvement in function occurs only when the system involved is challenged. Improvement occurs when, and only when, the workload is greater than that to which the individual is accustomed."[2] It should be stressed that overload is not the same as overwork. Overload involves placing enough stress on the body to stimulate the desired response without resulting in exhaustion.

7. *Progression is an important part of every exercise program.* The body will adapt to an increased level of resistance as improvement takes place. For this reason it is necessary to measure progress and to increase the work load frequently. It should also be emphasized that it is not wise to commence a vigorous program if one is accustomed to a sedentary way of life. The program should be moderate at first, and then progression will be incorporated as the body is able to adapt to the increased stress level. Students should not be discouraged by lack of progress at different times during the program. Progress is quickest and most apparent at the start of a program, particularly if the person has been inactive prior to the start of the program. Progress slows down as one approaches his maximal potential because, as progress continues, improvement becomes more difficult. It is only through increasing the workload that progression will be possible.

8. *A training program will result in specificity of improvement.* An exercise program is specific and will result in improvement only in the area or areas that it is designed to develop. For example, a person who lifts weights regularly will develop strength and muscular endurance only. Similarly, unless a person includes activities that involve large muscle groups and that result in heart rates exceeding 150 beats per minute for extended periods of time, he should

not expect to experience a notable improvement in cardiovascular endurance. The activities that make up the program will determine the results attained. The system adapts to the specific exercise attempted. A person who engages in walking becomes fit for walking, while a person who trains on a bicycle becomes a better bicyclist. A person who runs gets in shape for running. There is little carry-over from one activity to another.

FREQUENCY OF THE EXERCISE PROGRAM

Research indicates that a good exercise program should be performed at least four times per week and possibly not more than five times per week. Rest periods are essential and should be built into any exercise program. They result in both physical and mental relaxation.

LENGTH OF EACH EXERCISE SESSION

The length of each exercise session may vary according to the specific objectives. It appears that the proposed plan as recommended by the American Heart Association is adequate for most people. They suggest that each exercise session be divided into three segments as follows:

1. A 5- to 10-minute warm-up session so that the heart and circulatory system are not suddenly taxed.
2. A sustained 20- to 30-minute exercise series in which the heart rate remains in the target zone.
3. A 5- to 10-minute cool-down session in which the intensity of the task is lessened before exercise is stopped.

This plan is summarized in Fig. 13-1.

SELECTION OF ACTIVITIES

The reader is referred to Chapter 12 to determine which activities might be best for increasing the heart rate to the desired level. This will also depend upon the skill of the exerciser, the fitness level of the exerciser, the pattern of rest pauses, and the environmental temperature. It is

Fig. 13-1. Suggested exercise training pattern. (Courtesy Best Foods Division, CPC International, Englewood Cliffs, N.J.)

suggested that each person vary his program so as to maintain interest and motivation.

No matter which activities are selected, each person should check his heart rate as indicated above to make sure that the intensity is adequate to raise the heart rate to the desired level.

SEMESTER ASSIGNMENT

The laboratory assignment for the semester might include the development of a 3-month personal physical fitness program based on the individual needs of each student. The assignment should include the following:

1. A summary of the student's present physical fitness level. Each student should make use of the results of the tests that relate to physical fitness. These should be presented in a meaningful way with a conclusion concerning the student's present physical fitness level.

2. A statement of the objectives or goals that each student establishes for his physical fitness program. These should be presented in terms of student behavior and should state specifically what each student will be able to demonstrate if he successfully completes his program and attains the desired results.

3. Information relating to the activities included in the program. This section should include the following:

a. A list of activities.

b. The specific purposes for each proposed activity.

c. Samples of weekly schedules showing the amount of each exercise or activity. The samples should also demonstrate how progression is built into the program.

d. Procedures to be followed for evaluation of progress toward the desired goals.

REFERENCES

1. Cureton, T. K.: Run for your life. In The healthy life, New York, 1966, Time, Inc., p. 36.
2. DeVries, H. A.: Physiology of exercise for physical education and athletics, Dubuque, Iowa, 1966, Wm. C. Brown Company, Publishers, p. 218.
3. Hanson, D.: Health related fitness, Belmont, Calif., 1970, Wadsworth Publishing Co., Inc., p. 4.

ACTIVITY INVENTORY*

Now that you have completed this course, it is important to find out which activities you are actively engaged in and which ones you would like to learn more about.

Place a check mark in column 1 next to each activity that you have participated in regularly for at least 8 weeks any time during the past 12 months.

Place a check mark in column 2 next to each activity that you would like to learn more about and in which you would like to increase your skill level.

Numbers are included next to each activity so that computer cards may be used for tabulating results where desired. Students will use the number corresponding to each activity and make their responses next to that number on the IBM card.

Individual and dual sports

	Col. 1	Col. 2
1. Archery	☐	☐
2. Badminton	☐	☐
3. Bowling	☐	☐
4. Calisthenics	☐	☐
5. Fencing	☐	☐
6. Fly casting	☐	☐
7. Golf	☐	☐
8. Gymnastics	☐	☐
9. Handball	☐	☐
10. Hiking	☐	☐
11. Jogging	☐	☐
12. Judo	☐	☐
13. Paddleball	☐	☐
14. Skating	☐	☐
15. Skiing	☐	☐
16. Tennis	☐	☐
17. Track and field	☐	☐
18. Weight lifting	☐	☐
19. Wrestling	☐	☐

Dance

	Col. 1	Col. 2
20. Ballet	☐	☐
21. Ballroom	☐	☐
22. Creative	☐	☐
23. Folk	☐	☐
24. Square	☐	☐

Team sports

	Col. 1	Col. 2
25. Baseball	☐	☐
26. Basketball	☐	☐
27. Field hockey	☐	☐
28. Ice hockey	☐	☐
29. Soccer	☐	☐
30. Softball	☐	☐
31. Touch football	☐	☐
32. Volleyball	☐	☐

Aquatics

	Col. 1	Col. 2
33. Canoeing	☐	☐
34. Diving	☐	☐
35. Lifesaving	☐	☐
36. Sailing	☐	☐
37. Swimming	☐	☐
38. Water safety instruction (WSI)	☐	☐

Others (list)

	Col. 1	Col. 2
_____	☐	☐
_____	☐	☐
_____	☐	☐
_____	☐	☐

*Adapted from Humphrey, J. H., and Ingram, A. G.: Introduction to physical education for college students, Boston, 1969, Holbrook Press, p. 37.

ATTITUDE QUESTIONNAIRE

Now that you have completed this course, it is important to see what effect this class has had on your attitude toward exercise and physical education. Please respond to each of the following questions by placing a check mark in the appropriate column. Again you are asked to be honest and objective in your answers.

Age _____ Sex _____

Laboratory instructor _____

	Strongly agree	Agree	Undecided	Disagree	Strongly disagree
1. Little learning takes place in physical education classes.	☐	☐	☐	☐	☐
2. At the college level, physical education classes contribute little and do not justify the time and money spent on them.	☐	☐	☐	☐	☐
3. Physical education classes should be offered at the college level, but whether they are taken ought to be up to the students.	☐	☐	☐	☐	☐
4. Most information about exercise and physical fitness is common knowledge.	☐	☐	☐	☐	☐
5. Physical education should consist only of those activities that are fun to participate in.	☐	☐	☐	☐	☐
6. I would take physical education only if it was a university requirement.	☐	☐	☐	☐	☐
7. Physical education should develop in students an understanding of the importance of exercise to health and fitness.	☐	☐	☐	☐	☐
8. All required subjects at the college level in all areas except for the area that the student is majoring in should be offered only as electives.	☐	☐	☐	☐	☐
9. Most adults get all the exercise they need by performing their daily tasks.	☐	☐	☐	☐	☐
10. The development of an adequate level of physical fitness should be a worthwhile objective for all college students.	☐	☐	☐	☐	☐
11. This class contained little information of interest to me and was definitely a waste of time.	☐	☐	☐	☐	☐
12. All students at the college level should be exposed to such a course as this.	☐	☐	☐	☐	☐
13. I am now more active during my leisure hours than I was before I took this class.	☐	☐	☐	☐	☐

Index